ALTERNATIVE APPROACHES TO MEETING
BASIC HEALTH NEEDS IN DEVELOPING COUNTRIES

ALTERNATIVE APPROACHES TO MEETING BASIC HEALTH NEEDS IN DEVELOPING COUNTRIES

 A joint UNICEF/WHO study

Edited by

V. DJUKANOVIC
Chief Medical Officer

E. P. MACH
Technical Officer

Development of Health Services
Division of Strengthening of Health Services
World Health Organization
Geneva, Switzerland

WORLD HEALTH ORGANIZATION

GENEVA

1975

First impression, 1975

Second impression, 1976

ISBN 92 4 156048 7

PRINTED IN SWITZERLAND

CONTENTS

INTRODUCTION

Despite great efforts by governments and international organizations, the basic health needs of vast numbers of the world's people remain unsatisfied. In many countries less than 15% of the rural population and other underprivileged groups have access to health services. More serious still, these people are both particularly exposed and particularly prone to disease. A hostile environment, poverty, ignorance of the causes of disease and of protective measures, lack of health services or inability to seek and use them—all may combine to produce this sorry situation.

To meet the main health needs of the underprivileged, who make up about 80% of the population in less developed countries, health services should seek out these people, find what they need and want, and protect, treat and educate them. The strategy adopted for this purpose by many developing countries has been modelled on that of the industrialized countries, but as a strategy it has been a failure. The tendency has been to create relatively sophisticated health services staffed by highly qualified personnel, in the hope of expanding them progressively as resources increased until the entire population was covered. The outcome has been quite different. The services have become centred largely on the cities and towns, are predominantly curative in nature, and are accessible mainly to a small and privileged section of the population.

The relative emphasis on programmes to control specific diseases may also have hindered the development of basic health services over the past 25 years. As early as 1951, when the efforts of many developing countries were centred on specialized mass campaigns for the eradication of diseases, the Director-General of WHO pointed out in his annual report [a] that these efforts would have only temporary results if they were not followed by the establishment of permanent health services in rural areas to deal with the day-to-day work in the control and prevention of disease and the promotion of health.

The enthusiastic application of new knowledge and technology has not always achieved the results expected, and some of the consequences have been untoward. In sum, history and experience show that conventional health services, organized along " Western " or other centralized lines, are unlikely to expand to meet the basic health needs of all people. The human, physical and financial resources required would be too great and the necessary sensitivity to the special problems of rural or neglected communities would rarely be attained.

Clearly the time has come to take a fresh look at the world's priority health problems and at alternative approaches to their solution. This is not just a question of injecting a little more technical know-how. Some countries

---

[a] WHO Official Records, No. 38, 1952, p. 2.

7

will need to make drastic or revolutionary changes in their approach to health services ; others, at the very least, radical reforms. The remodelled approach must be linked to the prevailing human attitudes and values, which differ from community to community, and it will require a clear motivation and commitment on the part of the people who have the knowledge and the political and economic power to introduce change.

Background of the study

The magnitude and gravity of the problems, compounded as they are by widespread poverty, ignorance and lack of resources, are daunting. Nevertheless, much can be done to improve the health of the people in the developing world. In a number of countries successful or potentially successful programmes meeting basic health needs have been set up. They range from innovative programmes covering limited areas to completely new health systems introduced in the wake of radical changes in the political and social system—for example, in China, Cuba and, to a certain extent, Tanzania.

WHO and UNICEF decided to carry out a study of some of these new approaches in the hope that an analysis of them and of the shortcomings of conventional systems would enable the two organizations to develop fresh policies and approaches that could be reflected in their assistance to countries.[a] They realized that the study would not break new ground. The successful or promising approaches they examined are actual programmes, and some of them have already been studied and analysed.

The main purpose of the case studies described in Part II of this report was to single out and describe their most interesting characteristics and to enable them to be discussed openly and objectively. It is hoped that these discussions will encourage further studies and make the findings known to a wider public. The emphasis is not on further development of health services as they are now organized, but rather on new ways of identifying basic health needs and of providing simple preventive and curative health measures.

Objectives

Starting from the failure of conventional health services and approaches to make any appreciable impact on the health problems of developing populations, the study aimed at examining successful or promising systems of delivery of primary health care in order to identify the key factors in their

---

[a] The development of health service systems designed to meet basic health needs, particularly in the developing countries, is a subject of major concern for WHO and UNICEF ; within this context, UNICEF has a special interest in children's health, which is one of its overall goals. The past policies of the two organizations on basic health services are outlined in Annex 1.

success, and at observing the effect of some of these factors in the development of primary health care within various political, economic and administrative frameworks.

Particular interest was taken in features that appear to play a real part in improving basic health coverage, the mobilization of resources, the utilization of services, understanding of health problems and health services, the quality of health care, and the satisfaction of consumers and providers with the care given.

In this connexion, it was felt that an adequate approach to meeting basic health needs must provide, inter alia : sufficient immunization ; assistance to mothers during pregnancy and at delivery, postnatal and child care, and appropriate advice in countries that accept a family planning policy ; adequate safe and accessible water supplies, sanitation, and vector control ; health and nutritional education ; and diagnosis and treatment for simple diseases, first-aid and emergency treatment, and facilities for referral. Not all of those services need be provided together, but they should be planned purposefully as a gradual expansion. The approach should also be applicable, or promise to be applicable within a reasonable time in countries of very limited resources, and should seek to provide at least 80% coverage for such socially or geographically remote populations as villagers, nomads, and peri-urban and slum dwellers.

In the selection of new approaches for detailed study, emphasis was placed (a) on actual programmes that are potentially applicable in different sociopolitical settings, and (b) on programmes explicitly recognizing the influence on health of other social and economic sectors such as agriculture and education.

Methods

Information was gathered from a wide range of sources, including members of WHO advisory panels, publications, the reports of meetings, studies by UNICEF, WHO, the United Nations and other international agencies, and the WHO regional offices, country representatives, and field staff. On the basis of this information, promising programmes were selected and studied at the actual site by working teams with the full cooperation of the governments in Bangladesh, Cuba, India, Niger, Nigeria, Tanzania and Venezuela. Early in December 1973 a team of senior WHO staff visited China, and its observations were used in conjunction with an independent survey of the Chinese health system. On UNICEF's recommendation a project in Ivanjica, Yugoslavia, was included.

The study report was originally drafted by the authors (including the authors of the case studies) in consultation with a representative of UNICEF. The draft was reviewed and commented on by a group of WHO and UNICEF consultants at a meeting held in Geneva in June–July 1974.

9

The report was then redrafted and presented to the twentieth session of the UNICEF/WHO Joint Committee on Health Policy in February 1975.[a]

In May 1975, following its approval by the Joint Committee of the two organizations, the study was endorsed by the UNICEF Executive Board, which adopted its principles as UNICEF policy. Later in the same month the Twenty-eighth World Health Assembly considered the study, which was placed before it as a background document to serve as the basis for a major worldwide action programme for primary health care; this programme was approved by the Health Assembly in resolution WHA28.88.[b]

I. WORLD POVERTY AND HEALTH

What we know as the developing world, far from being a single homogeneous entity, is made up of a great variety of widely differing countries and areas at different stages of development. Nevertheless, their progress is conditioned by certain factors in common, and in some cases it may be possible to consider common solutions to their problems.

These problems have complex political, social, cultural, and environmental roots. Extremely limited resources, poor communications, vast distances, individual and community poverty, and lack of education act and react upon one another in such a way as to maintain the developing countries in a perpetual state of poverty.

The most obvious economic signs of underdevelopment are low labour productivity, a low national product, and a low average income per person. The standard of living in developing countries is low for the great mass of the people, and life is beset by the problems caused by insufficient or faulty food intake, poor housing conditions, poor health, inadequate public and private provision for hygiene and medical care, insufficient communication, transport, and educational facilities, and systems of education and training that are ill adapted to the people's needs.

Although, owing to such factors as different price systems and inflation, per capita income can be misleading as an index of the standard of living, it is worth noting that in some Asian and African countries the daily per capita income is about 20–24 US cents, and in some of them it is less than 6 US cents for the poorest 20% of the population. Per capita consumption in a number of countries is under US $94 a year. These figures compare starkly with an estimated per capita income in the USA of $4980 and in France of $3400 a year in 1972.

Low incomes defeat the desire of governments—which may be the only driving force able to introduce change—to provide public services, par-

---

[a] The study as it is now presented is a somewhat shortened version of that report.

[b] WHO Official Records, No. 226, 1975, p. 53.

ticularly social services, from national tax revenue for the poorest sector of the population.

Among the other obstacles to development, many countries have to contend with an unfavourable physical environment—poor soil, difficult terrain, lack of forest and mineral resources—and an adverse climate with periodic excessive rainfall, extremes of temperature, and droughts. These physical obstacles may be compounded by the insufficient or inappropriate application of modern science and technology and unfavourable international terms of trade.

The rapid increase in the world's population and its effect in defeating the efforts of developing countries to raise their standards of living have been emphasized often enough. In some developing countries it has more than cancelled out the increase in the gross domestic product, while per capita output has actually fallen.

According to estimates and projections for 1970–1980 in the United Nations *1970 Report on the World Social Situation*, the total population of the less developed regions may increase during the decade by 28%, the number of pre-school children by 21% and the number of school-age children by 28%. To provide this rapidly growing population with food, housing, education and employment, the developing world is faced with a task of daunting proportions. The challenge will become insuperable in the decades to come unless the present development strategy is radically changed.

The underprivileged

The rural population

In 1970, the rural population of the less developed regions of the world was estimated at 1910 million—75% of the total population. By the year 2000 it will probably have risen to 2906 million, despite wholesale migration from the country to urban areas.

At the same time, people in many rural districts are isolated and dispersed, so that public services of the conventional type, including health services, are difficult and expensive to provide. Isolation of a community from the outside world is bound to hamper communication and put a brake on the improvement of living standards. What is more, dispersal and isolation add to the difficulties of educating, training, and employing qualified manpower.

It is worth enumerating some of the characteristics of underdeveloped rural areas :

— economic stagnation

— cultural patterns that are unfavourable to development

- agricultural underemployment, and lack of alternative employment opportunities
- poor quality of life because of the scarcity of essential goods, facilities, and money
- isolation caused by distance and poor communications
- an unfavourable environment predisposing to communicable diseases and malnutrition
- inadequate health facilities and lack of sanitation
- poor educational opportunities
- social injustice, including inequitable land tenure systems and a rigid hierarchy and class structure
- inadequate representation and influence in national decision-making.

The nomads

There are some 50–100 million nomads and semi-nomads in the world. About 90% of them live in Africa or Asia, in the dry belt that circles the earth north of the Equator and includes the arid land from Senegal and the Sahel region of Africa through south-west Asia to Pakistan and India. In distinction to nomads, who depend on migration for their livelihood and have no fixed dwellings, semi-nomads, including transhumants, are periodic migrants with one or more fixed dwellings who often engage in some agricultural activity. Nomads usually keep domesticated animals—cows, camels, sheep, or goats—but some are hunters and collectors, as in Australia, the Kalahari desert, Amazonia, and the Arctic.

Nomads have their own needs and problems. As the present catastrophic drought in the Sahel region has shown, in nomadic life there is a narrow margin between survival and death. Because of their constant movement and dispersion, nomads are difficult to reach with health services, which tend as a result to neglect them. In some development plans they are ignored or wrongly included with the rural population. Their particular situation needs to be recognized and given separate attention.

Slums and shanty towns

During the last two decades there has been an enormous increase in the number of people living in slums and shanty towns in the poorer countries. This growth is continuing and perhaps accelerating. Today about one-third of city dwellers in the developing countries live in slums and shanty towns. The proportion is increasing and exerts a major influence on the city environment.

The main reason for this growth is that large numbers of people are moving from rural areas to the cities in search of work and a better life. This is not to say that work is easy to find in the cities. The urban population of developing countries is increasing much faster than the supply of jobs ; even so, the situation is worse in rural areas. Urban poverty is often a reflexion of the overflow of rural poverty.

Almost half the people now living in slums and shanty towns are children. At current growth rates, their number will double by 1980. This is the most tragic aspect of the problem—the slum conditions mortgage the future of many of these children, especially the very young in their most formative period of growth. Child mortality and suffering in these communities are very high and life expectancy is low.

The glaring contrasts in health

Throughout the world, for lack of even the simplest measures of health care, vast numbers of people are dying of preventable and curable diseases, often associated with malnutrition, or survive with impaired bodies and intellects. There are striking differences in the vital statistics for the under-privileged and the developed world. According to 1971 data, the life expectancy at birth was 43 years in Africa and 50 years in Asia, compared with 71 in Europe and North America.

During the last decade, maternal and childhood mortality rates have been steadily decreasing in most parts of the world. In many developing countries, however, the levels of mortality remain high and less progress has been made in reducing morbidity and improving the health and quality of life of mothers, children and families.

The most serious health problems of mothers and children and the high rates of mortality and morbidity in the world as a whole result from various interrelated conditions : malnutrition, infection, and the consequences of ill-timed, closely spaced, and too frequent pregnancies, and the lack of health care and other social services, against a background of generally poor social and economic conditions.

Problems related to the first year of life must be considered in the context of the 120 million or so births a year in a world population of more than 3400 million. According to United Nations estimates for 1965–69, some 84% of all births during that period occurred in developing countries. The estimated annual number of infant deaths in those countries over the same period reached 14.2 million out of 101 million live births, as compared with 516 000 out of 19 million live births in developed areas. In the less developed regions the infant mortality rate was 140 per 1000 live births, dramatically higher than the rate of 27 per 1000 in the more developed regions ; there was an enormous variation among countries, from an estimated maximum of about 200 to a minimum of 9.6 per 1000. If developing countries could bring their infant mortality rates down to the average rate of the developed, some 11 million infant lives could be saved each year.

For children aged one to four years, the death rate in general is relatively lower than for infants, but the contrast between developed and developing countries in this older age group is even greater. While on average the infant mortality rate is 10–20 times higher in developing than in developed countries, the average mortality rate between the ages of one and four years is 30–50 times higher.

Data on nutritional deficiency, low birth weight, and immaturity indicate that perhaps the single most important factor influencing the excessive mortality in developing areas is the deficient nutritional state of the population. Mothers who have been handicapped since early life by nutritional deficiency and various adverse environmental factors probably give birth to low-weight infants ; many of these infants die from infectious diseases because of their greater vulnerability, while those who survive continue, through nutritional deficiency, to be at higher risk from the hazards of the environment.

The principal causes of morbidity in the developing world are malnutrition, vectorborne diseases, gastrointestinal diseases, and respiratory diseases—themselves the result of poverty, squalor and ignorance. To them must be added the diseases of mothers related to deprivation, unregulated fertility, and exhaustion, with their effects on the unborn and newborn child. These conditions are linked with social problems such as overwork among women, unemployment among the young, population growth and urbanization ; and their solution calls for an integrated effort in which the health services have a major role to play.

The obstacles to be overcome

Remedies for many of the shortcomings of health services are known and available, but some cannot be usefully applied unless the overall concept of health care is appropriately modified. For a number of problems a new approach cannot in itself be considered a remedy, but rather as a prerequisite to the successful application of largely known remedial action. The main need today is to develop systems through which effective health care can be made both accessible and acceptable to the people.

Problems of broad choices and approaches

(a) *Lack of clear national health policies and poor linkage of health service systems with other components of national development*

An effective health approach requires the coordinated efforts of all those sectors that can contribute directly or indirectly to the promotion of wellbeing. This is so not only at the central level but also at the intermediate and—above all—the peripheral level, where policies should have their roots. Moreover, health should be considered as an integral part of development, with clearly defined goals, policies and plans. In many developing countries this approach is not followed. As a consequence, overall health goals and policies are missing, and this largely precludes health planning. The efforts made are fragmentary, not necessarily related to those of other sectors, and not directed towards supporting national growth on a broad scale by fostering human wellbeing and resources. Health activities often become stagnant and health development projects collapse for lack of proper budgetary support. Even when policies and goals are established and the principle of multisectoral action is accepted, agencies, either national or international, have difficulty in crossing sectoral lines in order to implement the decisions.

Measures have been developed, with the help of biomedical research, to tackle many of the health problems of developing countries. Although for some of the problems no simple and effective technology is available, many technologies have been standardized and simplified to such a degree that they can be used effectively at low cost and with inexpensively trained staff on a large enough scale to make a substantial impact. Regrettably, they are not yet being widely applied.

Much of modern health technology, however, is inappropriate or irrelevant to the immediate needs of people in developing countries. Moreover, owing to the high cost of sophisticated equipment and other requirements, it tends to absorb, for the benefit of a minority of the population, a substantial share of limited resources that should be used to benefit all the people. This is a problem that needs to be dealt with by national governments.

(b) *Lack of clear priorities*

Clear, concise and logical priorities within health care systems are rarely laid down. Realistic criteria for the development of priorities are formulated even more rarely. For example, scant attention is given to the balance between curative, preventive, and promotional activities and the division of resources among them ; curative services usually absorb a disproportionate share of money, manpower, and facilities. Priorities between primary care and referral care services are seldom defined in a general plan. Nor are priorities within the three main sectors themselves often clearly delineated. A balance is not always established on objective grounds between personal health services, environmental health services, and community-oriented activities. As a consequence, curative services and, more generally, personal services tend to receive undue emphasis, even when better results might be achieved by some other use of the same limited resources. Again, not enough is done to assess alternative methods of combating communicable diseases to obtain the best results, while the use of measures not directly related to but greatly affecting health is frequently neglected.

(c) *Opposition to changes in the social aspects of health policy*

The fact has to be faced that established health associations, institutions and organizations, particularly in the professional sphere, tend to resist changes such as the introduction of a national health service, compulsory or voluntary health insurance, or the employment of new categories of health manpower. Whatever the motives of these organizations—to defend their own interests or preserve cherished traditions—this resistance may have serious repercussions on health plans, programmes, and policies, since highly regarded members of the medical professions often have great influence on policy and on those who take the decisions, if they are not themselves the persons who make policy or take decisions.

(d) *Inadequate community involvement in providing health care*

Most health care delivery systems have failed to make care accessible and acceptable to the people who need it. Primary health care must be available close to people's homes. As the acceptance of many health measures may involve a change in living habits, the community itself must decide on the measures, help in carrying them out, and evaluate their success. Basic health care can be given by ordinary people provided they have adequate education, training, and technical advice and supervision.

It follows that there must be a clearly defined relationship between the two components of frontline health care—the activities carried out by the government and those carried out by the people themselves. The relative contribution of each of the two partners to health care activity as a whole should be determined by the political and socioeconomic situation in each country or geographical area.

Organizing the delivery of health care so that part of it " belongs " to those it is designed to serve has enormous advantages. Local resources can be tapped and the community's view of the nature of the system can be radically changed. Ideally, this component of health care delivery should be under the control and administration of the community itself, but such a division of responsibilities within the system need not detract in any way from the primary principle that health care delivery must be thought of and planned as a whole, in the light of clear goals for national health care.

The obstacles to community participation of this kind include :

— in some countries a political system that does not encourage local self-government—a prerequisite to local involvement in health and development in general

— the rigid sectoral structure and centralized organization of most conventional government health services

16

— competition between the traditional system of health care already existing at the local level and the modern system of health care

— the system of beliefs (religion, caste, etc.) of communities in peasant societies.

(e) *Inappropriate training of health personnel*

Education and training programmes, both undergraduate and post-graduate, at home or abroad, are frequently irrelevant to or fall short of local health needs and aspirations. Examples of educational systems planned to provide suitable staff for national health needs are few and far between. Graduates in general find it hard to adapt themselves to the type of work necessary to meet basic national needs and prefer to do the work they are trained for. Higher education thus tends to create a communication gap between professional personnel and primary health workers,[a] as well as between the professionals and the unsophisticated people they should serve. Professionals are in the main unwilling to work in the rural areas where health services are most needed while, paradoxically, they resist the delegation to nonprofessional health workers of responsibility for primary health care. The medical profession often opposes new types of health personnel on the ground that providing medical care is too important, too complex, and too dangerous to be left in the hands of less trained or differently trained personnel. This opposition may be disruptive since, in order to function effectively, primary health workers need the active support of physicians or other health service staff.

Equally, the training of auxiliaries today usually leaves much to be desired. Seldom is it planned according to priorities and the job to be done. More often the curricula look like simplifications of professional ones. To strengthen and add systematically to their professional knowledge and skills, in line with the national development plan for health services, auxiliaries with limited basic education and brief preparation require periodic refresher courses and more advanced training. They generally do not get them.

Problems of resources

(a) *Inadequacy and maldistribution of resources for health services*

The developing world lacks human, material, and financial resources to meet its health needs. In some countries there is an absolute shortage, and

---

[a] In this report, the term " primary health worker " is used for nonprofessional health personnel, including auxiliaries, who carry out frontline curative, protective and promotional work within health care delivery systems. Professional staff may also perform primary health care functions but will usually be referred to by their professional designation, e.g., physician, nurse, engineer.

the situation is often complicated by faulty utilization or distribution of the resources that exist.

Scarcity of money affects all parts of the health delivery system. It first shows itself at the national level, both in the routine allocation of yearly budgets to the various sectors of the economy and in the distribution of funds to authorities responsible for national development plans. One useful index of financial resources is per capita health expenditure; although this index is not strictly comparable among countries, the figure is low in all developing countries, and lowest in the neediest areas.

Though felt throughout the health system, the shortage of financial resources affects the larger, needier rural population more than the city dwellers. Frequently modelled on the pattern of the developed countries, the health sector of developing countries is often hospital-based, relies on relatively sophisticated technology, and places emphasis on specialized medicine. As a result, it may absorb an unduly large share of the health budget to serve a comparatively small, privileged clientele. In many developing countries over half of the national health budget is spent on health care in urban areas, the home of no more than a fifth of the total population.

The shortage and maldistribution of human resources are just as striking. The distribution of professional personnel within developing countries is almost inversely proportional to the distribution of the people. This phenomenon is not confined to physicians. Outside the main cities and towns there are very few professional health personnel, and they work in public, voluntary, or mission service. It is not uncommon for populations of 50 000 or even more to be served by one physician. Health personnel are also poorly distributed in most of the countries where a large number of professionals are trained. Most educational systems, as has already been suggested, produce professionals in accordance neither with the country's needs nor with the expectations of the trainees.

(b) *Non-utilization of actual and potential resources*

Despite the shortage of all types of resources, the paradoxical phenomenon of underutilization of the health services that are available is widespread in developing countries. The reasons for this differ from culture to culture and from situation to situation. In many cases it reflects such factors as the attitudes of health personnel, disregard of traditional systems and personnel, insufficient awareness of the need for community knowledge and involvement, physical and social inaccessibility, and poor transport. It is also true, however, that people are often not informed about available health services or are not clearly aware of the types of health measures offered or the reasons for them.

The " bypassing " phenomenon may also come into play; if people lack confidence in the local health institution they may ignore it, preferring when ill to go to urban hospitals or traditional practitioners. This leads to underutilization of health units and at the same time overburdens services, such as hospitals, that should more properly be providing secondary and not primary care. Initial studies indicate the considerable importance of this phenomenon, the consequence of inadequate service quality, failure to meet the community's expectations, staff arrogance, or discrimination. Other factors may be job dissatisfaction, exhausting workloads or unrealistic staffing, and inappropriate use of staff time.

Within the communities themselves resources lie untapped, ignored by today's designers of health services. They include the indigenous systems for providing health care—traditional birth attendants, midwives, healers and others, who work on a fee-for-service basis in many developing countries among large populations and are well established but unrecognized or inadequately recognized.

(c) *Restricted use of primary health workers*

One of the major obstacles to the development of health services in rural areas has been the absence of clear thinking about the kind of health personnel needed to provide the necessary services at the village level. Most preventive measures and a large number of medical procedures are simple and do not require extensive professional training. In recognition of this fact, there is now a trend towards establishing a body of primary health workers who can be trained more rapidly, less expensively and in greater numbers than doctors or nurses. It is particularly important to use them for primary care in rural areas.

Primary health workers can be recruited from among the villagers and be trained in or near the village, so that they truly belong to the people. They can be employed full-time or part-time.

However, the development of a system of primary health workers, while offering the promise of an alternative form of primary health care, may raise a new set of problems related to their selection and administration, their links with other parts of the health services, and their logistic support. For example, their generally limited basic education and short period of preparation require continuing on-the-spot training and the full support of the whole health service system. Existing health services have seldom provided training and support, nor have they wholeheartedly accepted the concept of utilization of primary health workers. Unless frontline workers have the backing of the rest of the health system, the rural populations may well reject a service that is clearly insufficient by itself.

Again, because primary health workers often work in remote areas without well developed communications and transport, it is difficult to ensure that they have the proper equipment and that patients can be easily referred to other levels of care. The remoteness of their posts also makes it more difficult to supervise and evaluate their work.

19

Other problems connected with the use of primary health workers are social. Traditional healers and medicine men may be antagonistic to these workers because they see them as a threat to their power and livelihood. Customs and taboos often militate against primary health workers, and problems arising from the traditional division of activities and prerogatives between the sexes also complicate the establishment of a new system.

So, although basically they may be willing to stay in the villages, primary health workers may be discouraged by the problems they face and prefer to move to the cities and better-paid jobs.

Critical importance attaches to the technical aspects of the activities of primary health workers, who form the entry point to the health system for the majority of the population. If they give the wrong treatment and do not refer patients when they should, the system will not function properly. And yet these individuals, the basic elements in the day-to-day functioning of the system, are the very ones who can receive only brief initial training. Consequently their tasks must be clearly defined and their training programmes must be efficient. The specification of tasks and the development of training programmes place a heavy burden on countries short of skilled manpower.

(d) *The rising cost of health services*

Rising costs in health care have recently been compounded by higher costs of basic commodities, fuel, and agricultural produce. The increasing cost of living, and particularly of food, is likely to aggravate the health problems of the vulnerable members of society and limit the ability of individuals and governments to pay for health services. The cost of medical programmes relying heavily on institutions and professional staff is increasing faster than that of simpler programmes. Obviously many economic factors are beyond the control of health decision-makers, but one measure well within their powers is to curb the growth of high-cost programmes and services for the few and promote low-cost services which, by using less expensive primary health care personnel, will reach a much larger proportion of the community. Such a measure must be accepted by the health establishment of all countries as a top priority and urgently needed change of direction.

Problems of the general structure of health services

(a) *Lack of effective planning machinery*

Although health planning has gained increasing currency in developing countries, for various reasons its implementation has not always been truly successful. The biggest weakness of many health planning endeavours is the lack of an overall health policy to guide them, of a political will to provide the resources necessary for implementation, and of an effective executive structure to implement the decisions. But there may be a host of other reasons for failure. Often health plans are not so designed that they can be integrated into the country's socioeconomic development programmes and planning is frequently focused on health services and not on meeting health needs. Information and effective machinery for national health planning are often lacking. Many health administrations are without competent planners, especially at regional level, or a planning system. The plans that are formulated are unrealistic, or not presented in terms attractive enough to appeal to the cost/benefit and cost/effectiveness minded economists of national planning bodies. This is a serious shortcoming, since planners and decision-makers tend to concentrate their attention on economic development, while social sectors, and health in particular, are relatively neglected. Another consequence is that plans are frequently directed towards intermediate objectives, some of which—prestige hospitals, training centres—are substantial and tangible but fail to achieve a change in the community's health status. Although this may seem an obvious step, the general population's needs, particularly at the local level, are not always identified before planning begins, and frequently the planning is based on statistical evidence that is either faulty or unrepresentative.

Behavioural scientists can make a considerable contribution to the planning and management of health, but their skills are little used. So, while social or psychological factors are often singled out as obstacles to solving health problems, action going beyond the admission of their importance is rare. In many cases the expectations of people, and particularly of rural people, are simply neglected, whereas they often reflect actual needs and satisfying them would go far towards gaining acceptance for measures to meet other needs not felt, but equally or more important.

(b) *Weak development of the " total system " concept*

Health care delivery systems—public and private, national and international, curative and preventive, peripheral, intermediate and central—must be considered as a whole.

In the health services, overcentralization of authority and executive responsibility may prevent effective and adequate delivery at the periphery. It tends to lead to an overconcentration of personnel, institutions and facilities, and so to the maldistribution of resources. Central authorities become too far removed from the bulk of the people and lose touch with community needs and expectations. Present systems of reporting seldom convey to the centre the full picture of requirements.

The integration of specialized programmes in the general health services is progressing, but slowly. While some programmes have been integrated, others remain largely autonomous. The fragmentation of a health service into disparate elements, each designed to serve a small section of the

21

population or a single purpose, militates against the goal of comprehensive and optimal utilization of limited resources. The trend is still to develop separate services, such as those for industrial health, school health, prison health and family planning, which would be better amalgamated into a single service.

The interaction between health services in the public sector and the remainder of the health system has not been fully studied or its importance appreciated. The non-public sector includes people and institutions with different levels of skill and resources, ranging from the specialized hospital to the private general practitioner, the pharmacist, the village midwife or even the local healer. All these services are part of the health care system, and national health authorities miss real opportunities by not taking advantage of the resources in the shape of money, manpower and local organization that already exist and can be directed towards national health goals. However, if the private sector is dominant, there is a danger that under-privileged sections of society will be deprived of essential health care, which should not depend largely on the purchasing power of the individual. It is therefore a national responsibility to provide health care that is free, or at least within the means of the individual. Most governments recognize this responsibility, but they often fail to find an approach that would progressively build up the community's capacity to provide such care—modestly at the beginning, if limited resources so dictate, but fairly to all their people.

Technical weaknesses

(a) *Inadequate health education*

High morbidity and high mortality, particularly among infants and children, are an index not only of a community's low health level but also of inadequate health education. A great number of diseases could be prevented with little or no medical intervention if people were adequately informed about them and if they were encouraged to take the necessary precautions in time. Prominent among these are most childhood diseases, nutritional diseases, especially during infancy, and diseases preventable by immunization. Health education is particularly needed where the network of services is weak ; there people must learn to protect themselves from disease and to seek help if they need it.

Efforts in health education have often been limited to giving information dogmatically, as if this alone would bring about a transformation. Inevitably, the outcome has been disappointing. The pattern of existing resources—economic, human and cultural—has been forgotten, and this too has contributed to health education's failure.

A nucleus of health education specialists may be necessary to plan and guide health information activities in a country, but it is surprising how much can be done by drawing on its frequently mentioned (and as frequently

22

ignored) human resources—the teachers, agricultural extension workers, community development agents and, depending on the culture, religious leaders, youth groups, traditional healers and so forth. There have been many instances of their effectiveness in educating the public, especially where illiteracy is prevalent, in the simple steps it can often take to prevent dangerous diseases. A field particularly suited to their efforts is environmental health, for example water sanitation and excreta disposal.

Health education can make a major contribution by giving people the self-respect derived from the knowledge that they can prevent disease and thus change the course of their life by their own efforts.

(b) *Lack of basic sanitation*

The quality of basic sanitation in most developing countries is well below the level considered necessary for the prevention and control of communicable diseases and the promotion and maintenance of physical, mental and social wellbeing. Basic sanitation should aim at safe water, a safe environment, uncontaminated food and a decent place to live. This demands good and sufficient safe water supplies, the sanitary collection and disposal of human wastes, the planning and control of urbanization, attention to proper housing, the control of pollution, food hygiene, vector control, and health education. The development of sanitation measures should be linked with economic and social development and community action. Modern concepts of basic sanitation are fairly new to many developing areas of the world. In addition, inertia permeates both the population and the officials responsible, who fail to grasp the need to initiate action. A major problem is often the lack of a competent service infrastructure to carry out a comprehensive range of functions efficiently.

A WHO survey in 91 developing countries revealed that only 29% of their total populations had access to safe drinking-water at the end of 1970. In urban communities 50% of the population obtained water through individual house connexions, while 19% used public standpoints. More than 85% of the rural population had no safe drinking-water available to them. Furthermore, many of the piped urban supplies functioned only intermittently, and so were potentially hazardous to health.

The immensity of the problem is illustrated by the relatively modest targets proposed for the Second United Nations Development Decade (1970–1980) : to provide 60% of the total urban population with a water supply in their homes and the remaining 40% with a water supply from public standposts ; to provide 27% of the urban population with sewer services; to provide 25% of the rural population with reasonable access to safe drinking-water and 10% with sanitary excreta disposal facilities.

The provision of basic sanitation for rural populations is a long-term undertaking on a vast scale, one that the health authorities cannot tackle alone. Quality standards and control are traditionally the responsibility of ministries of health. Other authorities—those concerned with agriculture, public works, mining and rural engineering, for example—may be better equipped to execute water supply and sanitation projects, and more acceptable to economic planners. This again calls for a multisectoral approach and close cooperation between government ministries or departments.

(c) *Deficiencies of communication and transport*

Health service systems cannot operate adequately without proper communication among their various elements, including the primary health workers in the villages. In most developing countries, many of the problems in the delivery of health services to rural areas are the consequence of poor transport and communications. They include insufficient supervision of the staff, lack of consultation and referral facilities, inadequate supplies of drugs and other health requirements, feelings of isolation and neglect among the staff, and a shortage of information about needs and possibilities.

Modern transport is not easily adapted to use in the developing world ; it has its own inherent problems, which are more acutely felt in countries without a technical orientation. Costs of operation are high in proportion to the countries' limited resources, technical understanding is often lacking at senior government level, and the skills to operate complicated machinery may be in short supply.

Since the late 1940s, UNICEF has given large numbers of various types of modern vehicle to support social service programmes. The delivery of these services has suffered because of failures in the transport component, and it is now recognized that if modern technical equipment is to be introduced and used in non-technically-oriented societies, guidance and training will be needed in the running of maintenance and repair services.

The 1970s have seen a more rapid increase in the cost of transportation than at any time in history, spurred by a dramatic rise in fuel prices. This increase has hit the developing countries proportionately harder than the developed countries and is now a major contributor to the rising cost of health services.

Developing countries with flying doctor services have also had to cope with many financial and technical difficulties. Moreover, these services are not usually designed to provide primary health care and appear to be effective only as a referral link where primary health care is available separately.

While many communication and transport problems may be solved by the use of two-way radio and aircraft, especially in specific conditions and for limited objectives as a component of some wider health service system, the cost per unit service is often exorbitant. Cost/benefit criteria have to be applied, the services being weighed against alternative methods of overcoming the problem of inaccessibility, including community involvement in primary health care to the point of self-sufficiency.

(d) Lack of adequate health information

Confusion between " statistical data " and " information " still reigns, with the result that many statistical services fail to provide public health administrators with the information they need for sound decision-making. If national systems are to be geared to solving the real problems of communities, a radical reform of objectives and methods of data collection is required. The routine collection of data of doubtful validity or utility serves neither the decision-makers nor the community ; on the contrary, it is a waste of resources that could better be spent on direct services to people. The value of routine data collection is open to question ; thoughtfully and intelligently planned, periodic sample surveys or reporting by exception may often provide more useful information at lower cost.

Information services should be recast according to the priorities of the health system and should be aimed strictly at problem-solving.

BIBLIOGRAPHY

BANERJI, D. *Health behaviour of rural populations*, New Delhi, Centre of Social Medicine & Community Health, Jawaharlal Nehru University, 1974.

BRYANT, J. *Health and the developing world*, Ithaca, Cornell University Press, 1969.

FENDALL, N. R. E. Auxiliaries and primary care. *Bull. New York Acad. Med.*, **48** : 1291–1300 (1972).

FENDALL, N. R. E. Primary medical care in developing countries. *Internat. J. hlth Serv.*, **2** : 297–315 (1972).

HARALDSON, S. S. R. Health problems of nomads. *Wld hosp.*, **9** : 176–177 (1973).

KESIC, B. Rural health problems and some aspects of their solution. *Israel Journal of Medical Sciences*, **4** : 544–552 (1968).

MYRDAL, G. *Asian drama : an inquiry into the poverty of nations*, New York, Pantheon, 1968.

NAVARRO, V. The underdevelopment of health or the health of underdevelopment : an analysis of the distribution of human health resources in Latin America. *Internat. J. hlth Serv.*, **4** : 5–27 (1974).

TAYLOR, C. E. & HALL, M. F. Health, population and economic development. *Science*, **157** : 651–657 (1967).

United Nations Department of Economic and Social Affairs. *A concise summary of the world population situation in 1970*, New York, United Nations, 1971 (Population Studies, No. 48), pp. 24–25.

United Nations Department of Economic and Social Affairs. *The determinants and consequences of population trends*, New York, United Nations, 1973 (Population Studies, No. 50), pp. 124–125, 135.

United Nations Department of Economic and Social Affairs. *World economic survey, 1969–1970*, New York, United Nations, 1971, p. 31 et seq.

United Nations Department of Economic and Social Affairs. *1970 Report on the world social situation*, New York, United Nations, 1971, pp. 146, 153.

United Nations Department of Economic and Social Affairs. *Statistical Yearbook 1973*, New York, United Nations, 1974.

United Nations Department of Economic and Social Affairs. *Demographic Yearbook 1973*, New York, United Nations, 1974.

United Nations Economic Commission for Africa. *World plan of action, African regional plan for the application of science and technology to development*, Addis Ababa, 1973.

UNICEF. The child and the city. *UNICEF News*, No. 77, 1973.

UNICEF. *The young child : approaches to action in developing countries*, New York, 1974 (unpublished UNICEF document No. E/ICEF/L.1303).

UNICEF/WHO Joint Committee on Health Policy, sixteenth session. *Assessment of environmental sanitation and rural water supply programmes assisted by the United Nations Children's Fund and the World Health Organization (1959–1968)*, Geneva, World Health Organization, 1969 (unpublished document No. JC16/UNICEF-WHO/69.2).

UNICEF/WHO Joint Committee on Health Policy, eighteenth session. *Assessment of UNICEF/WHO assisted education and training programmes*, Geneva, World Health Organization, 1971 (unpublished document No. JC18/UNICEF-WHO/2).

WHO Official Records, No. 225, 1975 *(Fifth report on the world health situation, 1969–1972)*, Part II.

WHO Official Records, No. 206, 1973, Annex 11 *(Organizational study on methods of promoting the development of basic health services)*.

WHO Meeting of Regional Advisers in Environmental Health. *Report*, Geneva, 1973 (unpublished WHO document No. EH/73.12).

II. MAIN FEATURES OF THE CASE STUDIES

The case studies presented in this chapter were selected on the basis of recommendations from members of WHO expert advisory panels and from WHO regional offices, and of information found in various documents, reports and publications. The programmes described here are only some examples of innovations in different parts of the world. Many of the programmes cannot yet be considered as successful, but only as promising attempts. The studies belong to three main categories. The first consists of innovative health care programmes introduced at the national level. The second category contains examples of promising health care action of limited range. The third consists of examples of programmes with a potential for extension or improvement of health services coverage.

The cases are described, together with some background information, in this part of the report. Full reports on each case, including further details on the country or area and on the programme, are available as separate documents, often with annexes describing particular features. Readers wishing to study the programmes in detail are referred to these full-length reports.[a]

---

[a] Available on request from the Division of Strengthening of Health Services, World Health Organization, 1211 Geneva, Switzerland.

Bangladesh: Approach to the development of health services[a]

General characteristics

The country, which occupies some 142 450 km^2, is divided into 19 districts and over 400 *thanas*.[b] The estimated population is now 75 million: 85% of the people live in rural areas, and the rest in 68 towns and cities.

The per capita income in 1973 was US $58 per annum, that for the poorest 20% of the population US $20.

Basic health conditions and health care policies

(a) *Pattern of diseases*

Infectious diseases are the most important causes of morbidity and mortality. Malaria, tuberculosis, smallpox, cholera and other diarrhoeal diseases and children's diseases such as diphtheria, neonatal tetanus, whooping cough and measles are still major problems. The malaria eradication programme has effectively reduced this disease except in border areas. There are about 100 000 deaths annually from pulmonary tuberculosis and 300 000 tuberculosis patients require hospital treatment. The prevalence of tuberculosis in industrial workers ranges from 2.6% to 4.5%. The smallpox epidemic in 1971 took a considerable toll—2510 cases were reported in the first four months. About 6% of the population bear pockmarks on the face, denoting previous smallpox infection. Cholera is endemic in the country and there is an urgent need for safe water supplies and hygienic disposal of human excreta.

(b) *General orientation of health services system before independence*

In the past there was a tendency to launch single-purpose programmes to solve individual public health problems. Such programmes have the following drawbacks:

1. They are self-limiting in the sense that as soon as the goal is achieved the programme is stopped or maintained only in skeleton form. Because of the lack of secure career prospects, it is difficult to attract dedicated workers of good quality.

---

[a] Visit made and case study prepared by Professor A. Akbar (UNICEF), Dr R. H. O. Bannerman (WHO), Dr V. Djukanovic (WHO), and Dr U Ko Ko (WHO).

[b] A *thana* is a police district usually containing 100 000–200 000 people. Each thana is divided into " unions " of about 15–20 villages.

2. There is duplication of effort, expenditure and trained personnel in the various programmes.

3. Some of the projects have a lopsided staff structure, with a concentration of technical and supervisory personnel at the centre.

4. Financial allocations to single-purpose projects are sometimes grossly disproportionate to the actual needs. While there are liberal allocations to some programmes, so that funds are unused or even wasted, other programmes cannot operate because of the shortage of funds.

(c) *Strategy for development of health services after independence*

The basic strategy in Bangladesh is to shift the emphasis from curative to preventive health care so as to bring the two into balance, and to develop a delivery system that provides integrated and comprehensive health care for the rural population. To achieve this, a rural health complex comprising rural health centres and 25-bed hospitals with satellite subcentres is established at each *thana*. Referral services for the rural health complex are provided through the subdivisional and district hospitals and other teaching and specialized institutions.

The emphasis in the health care delivery system has been shifted from the individual to the community, whose basic unit is the family. Thus it has become imperative to understand the ecology of the community and the development process as it affects education, agriculture, and economic progress, priorities and planning. The Government's policy requires a multisectoral approach and planning not just of the health services but for the health of the people. Health services are therefore based on integrated and comprehensive community health care covering all social and economic activities.

The objectives of Bangladesh's health policy are as follows :

1. To create a health infrastructure in the rural areas providing integrated and comprehensive health services through *thana* health complexes and union subcentres.

2. To integrate the family planning and health programmes at the grassroot level under the leadership of the *thana* health administrator so as to prevent as many unwanted pregnancies and births as possible.

3. To provide a well-organized health care programme for infants, children and mothers by strengthening maternal and child health services, with a view to reducing infant and maternal mortality.

4. To ensure effective control or eradication of communicable diseases and to organize epidemiological services supported by well-equipped public health laboratories.

5. To establish well-organized industrial health services for industrial workers, to provide protection against industrial health hazards, to create a healthy environment at places of work, and to provide workers and their families with medical care.

6. To improve the quality of existing hospital facilities, to provide new hospital facilities (with major emphasis on the establishment of at least one 25-bed hospital in each rural *thana*), and to reach the target of one hospital bed per 3500 population by the end of the plan period (1973/74–1977/78).

7. To create adequate undergraduate and postgraduate teaching and training facilities for medical, auxiliary, nursing and midwifery personnel and to ensure proper service conditions enabling the staff to be used to the optimum extent.

8. To ensure the availability of life-saving drugs for the treatment of the sick and of immunizing agents for the prevention or control of communicable diseases.

9. To ensure intersectoral cooperation and coordination in improving environmental sanitation, housing, potable water supply, etc., at home and work for every citizen.

(d) *General health service structure*

The rural health complex provides integrated and comprehensive health and family planning services for the rural population. Each rural health complex has two components : (i) a rural health centre at the *thana* level and subcentres at the union level ; (ii) a 25-bed hospital at the *thana* level.

The intention is to provide one rural health centre in each of the 356 rural *thanas* and one subcentre in each of 3698 rural unions. Each union subcentre will cover a population of approximately 12 000–15 000. The establishment of these health centres and subcentres is being spread over several years, according to the resources and manpower available.

Auxiliaries, called basic health workers, are key members of the health team. Basic health workers are educated to matriculation level and given special training. Each is in charge of not more than 4000 people and has adequate supervision. Basic health workers make regular home visits according to a planned schedule within a delineated area and each family is visited at least once a month.

During their home visits, they perform the following functions :

1. Immunization—primary vaccination and revaccination against smallpox, cholera and typhoid ; BCG vaccination.

2. Health education on environmental sanitation, water purification and family health, including family planning.

3. Collection and transmission to the rural health centre laboratory of blood samples of suspected malaria cases and sputum samples in suspected tuberculosis.

4. Supply of antimalarial, antituberculosis and antileprosy drugs to confirmed cases.

5. Participation in programmes against malaria and other epidemic diseases.

6. Maintenance of family health and family planning cards (through which vital statistics and other health and family planning data will be collected).

Basic health workers come under the supervision of an assistant health inspector, who is in charge of four basic health workers at union level and is in turn supervised by the medical officer or medical assistant in charge of the subcentre. In addition, every subcentre at union level has a maternal and child health clinic with family planning services under a lady health visitor.

The medical officer or his assistant functions as the team leader and is responsible for integrated health care for the entire union. Wherever necessary, he refers cases to and seeks help and guidance from the *thana* health administrator, who is his supervisor. At *thana* level the rural health centre is the headquarters for the integrated health services provided in the entire *thana* through its union subcentres. In addition to serving the union in which the *thana* health centre is situated, it provides leadership and referral services for all subcentres through its 25-bed hospital.

By early 1974, some 12 500 basic health (or family welfare) workers had been retrained and were functioning effectively ; it was planned to achieve full coverage of the population by basic health workers by the end of that year. The Government intends to set up a permanent training system to improve the knowledge and skills of the basic health workers and the quality of the care they provide.

(e) *Conclusion*

The reorganization of the health services, through reorientation and retraining of health personnel and the integration of health workers' functions, has reduced duplication of health activities and greatly improved health care delivery. More effective coverage of health care, particularly in the rural areas, has been achieved through the introduction of basic or primary health workers (called family health workers), who make monthly visits to homes to perform simple, well-defined tasks for health protection and promotion. In Bangladesh, where much of the terrain is waterlogged and communications are difficult, a relatively simple system of health care delivery of the type described above appears to hold the most promise.

The Savar project

(a) *General orientation*

A group of Bangladesh health workers organized the Savar project during the struggle for independence in line with the general strategy for the development of health services. The approach fits into the Government's present plan for a base unit (primary health centre) serving a network of subcentres.

The emphasis of the programme is largely preventive; it concentrates on immunization against communicable diseases and the development of family planning services. Limited curative services are available through clinics at the base and the subcentres. Inpatient facilities and emergency services are provided at the base hospital.

One of the project's basic principles is that health care cannot be viewed in isolation but rather as a part of overall development. Members of the community are taught handicrafts and improved agricultural methods to increase their family income. Health education is given in conjunction with the agricultural and nutrition programmes. A full-time education extension officer is in charge of the centre—officially known as the Bangladesh hospital and rehabilitation centre—with two teaching assistants.

The intention is that the Savar project should be as nearly self-supporting as possible by relying on insurance subscriptions from the population. For a monthly fee of 2 takas [a] per family, insured persons receive free outpatient treatment, and when hospital admission is necessary they pay an extra fee of 5 takas and one taka a day. No food is provided for inpatients but all medicines are free. Persons not covered by insurance pay 2 takas per visit but receive free medicine, and admission to hospital has to be paid for.

(b) *Description of the project*

Started in 1972, the project seeks to provide comprehensive health care for a population of over 200 000 in Savar *thana*, a rural area of 345 km². With a small hospital as the referral base, it is planned to establish a network of 11 subcentres, through which primary health care is to be delivered by locally trained village health workers backed by weekly visits to the hospital by a doctor. The headquarters are in Savar, and a daily clinic and emergency services are provided.

The Savar project is a service/training programme. In certain areas doctors visited the schools and selected volunteers from students. The aim was to recruit two students from each village and train them to provide preventive services in the village, mainly vaccination. This training programme is now being carried out. When they have completed their 6 months'

---

[a] 1 taka = US $0.12 (1974).

training, the students are expected to provide curative treatment for minor ailments, health education, and family planning advice. Village women are also trained and used to spread the family planning message ; they provide advice and family planning material. Trainees are given some remuneration for their services.

Students from the university and schools are being organized for medical social work, including adult education. All the villages are being surveyed and the necessary documentation, prepared by trainees or voluntary workers from schools and colleges, is checked by the doctors during visits.

A unique aspect of the programme is a self-insurance scheme under which outpatient treatment on three days of the week, emergency care at any time, drugs, immunizations and family planning services are provided for subscribers in return for a very modest monthly contribution. Although the amount thus paid directly by the consumer for these health services is small and poses no financial hardship, the originators of the scheme point out that it is more than double the amount that the Government is now able to spend per family on *all* health services in Bangladesh. The project began with virtually no funds, in spite of which it has functioned with remarkable effectiveness.

(c) *Economic support for health services*

The Savar project aims to be as nearly self-supporting as possible, by relying on insurance subscriptions. Four out of the 11 unions in Savar are initially to be covered by the insurance programme. The total population of these four unions is 60 000, of whom 50% have accepted the insurance scheme.

The chief criticism of the Savar project is that it is receiving a great deal of outside aid and there is doubt whether or not it will be self-sufficient in the near future.

(d) *Project administration*

Control of the hospital and rehabilitation centre is vested in an autonomous board of trustees, comprising two permanent representatives of the Bangladesh Medical Association and three eminent social workers. The management of the hospital is the responsibility of a board of governors, who elect the project director and administer the hospital under the plans and budget approved by the trustees. The board of governors consists of representatives of each of the major categories of hospital staff (physicians, nurses, administrators, etc.), together with a representative of the Bangladesh Medical Association, the Red Cross, and the faculty and students of the *thana*'s one university.

(e) *Community participation*

Although only a fraction of the cost of the services is met by insurance subscriptions, direct participation in the provision of their own health care has already produced a distinct change in the attitude of the villagers towards the health services, which have come to represent value for money rather than a public dole.

Since the overall programme is described by its founders as a "health and welfare scheme", an effort has also been made to provide employment for the consumers of the health services. One of the more successful activities has been the establishment of a sewing centre, where women are taught the use of sewing machines for the production of simple articles of children's clothing, for which they are paid on a piecework basis. The garments are then sold at a nominal price to the poorest families in the insurance scheme. A more important aspect of the sewing centre, however, is the opportunity it gives to offer the women a basic education and to encourage their participation in the health and family planning programme.

(f) Conclusion

Care must be exercised in deriving conclusions from the Savar project, because it has been in operation for a relatively short period and has had extensive outside support from the start. Moreover, the Savar region is probably not as poor as most of Bangladesh. However, several important inferences can be drawn :

1. It is possible and desirable for medical practitioners to be leaders in the institution of a radically different health system provided the effort is consistent with the national philosophy.

2. At least a partial self-insurance scheme will work even in extremely poor areas, provided there is a reasonable degree of financial security or stability. Financial security can be created for farmers through crop insurance schemes, but this requires huge financial involvement on the part of the government, particularly in a country such as Bangladesh where floods and cyclones are common.

3. Contributions from individuals for health care remove the stigma of charity and create an awareness of the value of health in the mind of the contributors. This is an important achievement. The creation of health awareness is a keystone in the development and planning of community health care programmes.

Savar provides a good example of a training programme for school and college student volunteers for the provision of preventive and curative services to rural populations in their own villages. It has been shown that adult education and vocational training programmes can be incorporated in a project that both improves health education and helps to increase the per capita income.

Jurain nutrition project

(a) *Background*

The Jurain project is in many ways similar to the Savar project, but it is based on local self-help without any external aid. The project was conceived by the President of the Diabetic Association of Bangladesh, who recognized that a nutrition project offers a good opportunity for field study of the community's socioeconomic and health status.

In a baseline nutrition survey conducted in 1964, 50% of the population were stated to be malnourished, and 75% of the children had protein-calorie insufficiency with clinical manifestations of vitamin A and vitamin B deficiency. In 1968 a pilot study was therefore initiated in Jurain, a suburb of Dacca, to find ways of improving the nutritional status of the population, mainly through self-help. Health education was attempted and the community was encouraged to increase its consumption of vegetables, fruit, fish, poultry, eggs, milk and wheat by cultivating hitherto unused arable land, raising poultry and rearing rapidly multiplying fish.

Baseline data were collected during the first year and a census was organized in the demonstration zone, which consisted of some 900 houses and 4000 inhabitants. Family status, nutrition and dietary habits, and educational levels were recorded. The amount of land available for farming and the number of livestock were also noted. Among the inhabitants, 80–90% were stated to have helminthic infections—mainly hookworm and roundworm.

(b) *Action programme*

A complex of bungalow-type houses was constructed at Jurain and the following action programme was instituted :

1. A farming centre was established where modern farming methods are demonstrated. Vegetables are grown and poultry and cows are reared under the supervision of an agricultural officer.

2. A women's centre was established to cater for the social needs of the women in the community. Here they are taught to knit and sew dresses, to make jute handicrafts, and to cook (through practical demonstrations).

3. A health centre was set up, with priority for women and children. Prenatal and postnatal clinics are conducted ; they include infant welfare and family planning among their services.

4. A youth centre was established and is responsible for adult education classes. Special instruction is given on modern agricultural practices, and young people are encouraged to take up farming.

34

(c) *Effects of the project*

In the third year a review of activities showed that the proportion of households with kitchen gardens had increased from 4% to 84%. Many were also rearing poultry and vaccinating their poultry and cattle periodically. A total of 46 ponds and ditches had been stocked with young fish.

Dietary habits had also been influenced favourably and green vegetables, previously eschewed by the community, had become an acceptable dietary item. The consumption of protein foods such as meat, fish and eggs showed a considerable increase.

The dietary habits of pregnant women and children had also been favourably influenced, with a considerable improvement in weaning practices. All pregnant women in the demonstration zone were encouraged to attend the prenatal clinic at least once during pregnancy ; such visits were an unusual occurrence in that community.

Poor environmental conditions were responsible for a high incidence of communicable diseases such as gastroenteritis, skin infections and respiratory diseases. In order to improve environmental sanitation, tube wells and latrines were constructed for the community. The population was inoculated against smallpox, cholera and typhoid, and children were being immunized against diphtheria, tetanus and whooping-cough.

It was reported that there had been no outbreak of cholera or smallpox in the area for three years.

(d) *Conclusion*

This project demonstrates clearly how the quality of life can be raised appreciably through the people's own efforts—environmental sanitation being improved by simple procedures and nutrition by more effective agricultural practices, and maternal and child health and social services being provided for hitherto illiterate and non-productive women in the community. In addition, the project shows that it is possible to obtain local support for activities that will improve the health of a community.

Health care in the People's Republic of China [a]

National policies

Over the past quarter-century, the People's Republic of China has fundamentally reorganized the politics, economy, and administrative services—including health services—of the world's most populous country. In a country only a short time ago ravaged by starvation and communicable disease and possessing extremely limited personnel and facilities for modern medicine (and those few concentrated in urban areas), a radical and rapid

---

[a] Case study prepared by Ruth Sidel and Dr V. W. Sidel.

change has been achieved. The principles on which the successful revolution (called in China the Liberation) in 1949 were based include. :

1. The redistribution of resources and of the power to allocate them from a small élite to a mass base, while preserving many basic cultural and national values.

2. A commitment to the development of services, including medical services, for those who previously had least—in the Chinese expression, the " workers, peasants and soldiers ".

3. An emphasis, especially since 1966, on the provision of services in the rural areas, where 80–85% of the Chinese people live.

4. A policy of developing these services as much as possible through local self-reliance and the involvement of all the people in a community rather than through the supply of services from higher levels or through highly trained personnel. This decentralization and use of personnel trained for very short periods is part of a highly organized and disciplined system of services.

5. A recognition of the value of traditional Chinese medicine, particularly in the rural areas, and its integration with what the Chinese call " Western medicine ".

6. An emphasis on preventive medicine and its implementation through mass campaigns and through association with therapeutic medicine of both the Western and traditional Chinese type.

7. The instillation of new social attitudes into health professionals and the reduction of the social distance between health workers and the people they serve. This is combined with opportunities for health workers at all levels to move to more complex levels of work through further training and experience.

8. Motivation through a sense of devotion to the community and to China as a whole ; a belief in people's ability to change and improve, given the appropriate education and environment ; and an ethic that views " serving the people "—rather than personal advancement—as the highest good to which all should aspire.

Development of health services

Although attempts were made at national health planning in the 1930s and 1940s through a national health administration, the then Government of China was unwilling or unable to develop services for the vast bulk of the population. The programmes were often barely relevant to and barely scratched the surface of the community's needs.

In the " liberated " areas, first in Kiangsi Province in the late 1920s and early 1930s and, after the Long March, in and around Yenan in Shensi

Province in the late 1930s and the 1940s, health services had high priority and were developed very differently. The basic principle followed was to involve the people themselves in the development and shaping of their own services through a process of discussion, questioning, criticism, and self-criticism. Although central policy direction, advisers, and some resources provided by the Army existed, each area made its own decisions and provided its own resources and manpower.

After the Liberation in 1949 a national health congress in Peking established four basic principles for health work : serving the workers, peasants, and soldiers ; putting prevention first ; uniting doctors of both traditional and Western medicine ; and integrating public health work with mass movements.

At first the Chinese Ministry of Health developed along organizational lines similar to those of the USSR Ministry of Health, and it apparently used similar strategies. For example, the first five-year plan (1953–1957) stated :

> " In developing health and medical services, priority must be given to improving the work in industrial areas, in areas where capital construction is in progress, and in forest areas, and sanitation work in rural districts must be gradually improved " (1).

This wording suggests an early policy emphasis on urban industrial areas, lower priority being given to services for rural areas.

Manpower policies were also similar to those adopted in the USSR. Higher medical education was vastly expanded, and a standard six-year curriculum with separate faculties for adult therapeutic medicine, paediatrics, public health, and sanitation was introduced.

The number of doctors rose from approximately 20 000 (1 : 25 000) to 150 000 (1 : 5000) between 1949 and 1965. Large numbers of middle-level health workers—170 000 assistant doctors (similar to the Soviet feldshers), 185 000 nurses, 40 000 midwives, and 100 000 dispensers—were also trained (2). This extraordinarily rapid production of newly trained health workers made a great difference in the availability of care, but their number was still far too small and their concentration in the cities still too great to meet the need.

At the same time large numbers of new hospital beds were built, raising the number from some 90 000 (1 : 6000) in 1949 to some 700 000 (1 : 1000) in 1965. In 1965 a Ministry of Health official reported that each of China's 2000 counties had at least one hospital (3), and other centres of excellence were established. However, one bed per 1000 population was still thought far too little for adequate care and the centres were too limited and too few.

At the same time the Government was fostering developments directed toward mass participation. Through the patriotic health campaigns sanitation was improved and pests such as flies and mosquitos were largely wiped out. Opium addiction was brought to an end and venereal diseases were essentially eliminated by campaigns conducted by locally recruited and briefly trained workers with community support. Vast numbers of people participated in campaigns against schistosomiasis and other parasitic infestations. Mobile health teams brought some measure of preventive medicine to isolated areas. Limited experiments were tried, particularly at the time of the Great Leap Forward in 1957–1959, in the local development of medical care, the provision of mobile medical care teams, and the training of what later came to be known as " barefoot doctors ".

In spite of these significant advances in professional manpower and facilities and in mass efforts, and demonstrable results in, for example, the reduction of the incidence of communicable disease and infant mortality rates, there was considerable criticism of the Ministry of Health in the mid-1950s on a number of grounds. Although there had been some success in redistributing resources to the rural areas, urban health services still received a disproportionately large share. With 80% of the population living in the countryside, the disproportion was glaring. Some programmes in preventive medicine had achieved striking success, but curative medicine still predominated in research, teaching, and health services. Moreover, traditional medicine received relatively short shrift and enjoyed a low status compared with " scientific " medicine.

Despite recognition of the importance of modifying techniques borrowed from other countries to fit China's unique conditions, much of medical education, public health, and medical care administration introduced into China from 1949 to the early 1960s was copied directly from Soviet models. It was realized that collective leadership and the use of education and persuasion were needed to implement policies, but a hierarchical managerial structure had developed, the top of which was said to be relatively unresponsive to criticisms or suggestions from the bottom. Though the first requirement was to ensure that everyone had access to the limited medical resources, there was increasing concern with the raising of standards rather than popularization of what was already available. It was said, for example, that the number of health workers of the barefoot doctor type trained and used near Shanghai was reduced in the early 1960s in the name of quality.

Finally, and perhaps most important of all in the eyes of the Chinese leadership, although managers were required to keep in touch with those they served and the tradition of valuing intellectual work more highly than manual work had been rejected, these principles of Chairman Mao appeared in some ways to be honoured more in the breach than in the observance.

In June 1965, foreshadowing the Cultural Revolution, Chairman Mao Tse-tung criticized the Ministry of Health for its lack of attention to rural areas in its service programmes and six-year medical course, for its emphasis on theoretical knowledge in the training of physicians, and for its lack of attention to the prevention and treatment of common diseases in research. He concluded his statement : "In medical and health work, put the stress on the rural areas ! " In response to this directive, and to the Great Proletarian Cultural Revolution of 1966–1969, many of the classical methods were at least temporarily abandoned. Much of the apparatus of the Ministry of Health was dismantled and it and its purposes were subjected to the "struggle, criticism, and transformation" that marked many Chinese institutions during the Cultural Revolution. Higher and middle medical school education was interrupted and did not resume until 1971, and then in a markedly shortened and modified form. Publication of medical and research journals was suspended until 1973.

The classic technical models were replaced by a much more vigorous attempt at the popularization of medical services. Mobile medical teams had visited remote rural areas in the past, but during the Cultural Revolution they expanded greatly in number, duties, and areas covered. All urban medical workers were required to spend a period in the rural areas, so that at any given time one-third of urban personnel were out of the cities and some moved permanently to the countryside. One million barefoot doctors and 3 million rural health aides were trained. Local cooperative medical care systems were developed and expanded in both rural and urban areas. In 1974, although medical education and medical journals had resumed, there remained aspects of decentralization and deprofessionalization that appeared to result directly from the Cultural Revolution.

Medical care in rural areas

The territory of China covers 9 598 281 km². The precise population is unknown, but current estimates are in the neighbourhood of 800 million, making it by far the world's most populous country. Eighty to 85% of China's population lives in its rural areas, but the population is unevenly distributed ; the vast majority of the people live in eastern China, and western China is exceedingly sparsely populated (4).

Up to 1949 China's land was largely concentrated in the hands of a relatively small number of landlords. It was estimated in 1937 that almost two-thirds of China's farmers rented land from others, and were forced to pay heavy rents. These poor peasants, who often worked land owned by absentee landlords with little concern for the peasants' conditions, received neither an adequate remuneration for their toil nor an adequate share of the food they produced (5). Repeated cycles of drought and flood added to the uncertainty and misery, so that even the peasants who worked their own small plot could be destroyed by a few bad crops.

One of the first priorities in each liberated area was for the peasants themselves to distribute the land among those who worked and lived on it (6). In the period following the Liberation the land and the primitive tools for working it thus became the property of individual peasants.

During the 1950s collective ownership increased and cooperatives were formed. By the late 1950s, as part of the Great Leap Forward, much of the farmland had been converted into communes, with collective ownership of agricultural tools and of the land, except for small private plots on which the peasants could grow food for personal consumption. The communes were often large enough to include all the households of a township, whose government was then combined with the management of the commune. Unlike the cooperatives, which were purely economic organizations, the communes became units of both political and economic organization. Their representative assemblies function as the townships' " people's congresses ". Today communes are formal, self-contained political units with their own internal government, usually reporting directly to the government of the county in which they are situated. There are now some 27 000 communes in China, with populations of up to 60 000.

The smallest subdivision of the commune is the production team, with a membership of 100–200 people. The team leadership is responsible for the day-to-day planning of the team's work. People in the same production team live close to one another, usually in small villages, and form the basic social unit in the countryside. A group of teams, usually some 10–20, combine to form a production brigade, which usually has wider responsibility than the team for health, transportation and, in the north, the grinding and storing of grain and has become the basic economic unit for the distribution of income to the peasants. A typical commune is composed of 10–30 production brigades. The commune is the lowest level of formal state power in the rural areas, analogous to the " neighbourhoods " in the cities, and is responsible for overall planning, education, health and social services, and the operation of small factories that produce goods for its members and for outside distribution.

China's rural health services at each level (outlined in Table 1) are summarized below. Health care for the production teams is provided by barefoot doctors and, in some areas, by part-time volunteer health aides who deal with problems of sanitation under the supervision of the barefoot doctors. The barefoot doctors provide medical care, including health education, prevention, and the treatment of minor illnesses, in their sparsely furnished health stations, which are located in the production team area within easy walking distance of the peasants' homes. They also provide care in the fields, taking their medical bag with them when doing agricultural work. The production teams also choose health aides, whose primary role is to teach people about sanitation, to collect night soil, and to ensure that it is stored for 10 days in cement vats before being used as fertilizer. The health aides work in their lunch hour or after their regular work and are not paid for this duty.

Health facilities at the brigade level vary widely in different parts of China. The care at this intermediate level is again provided by barefoot

TABLE 1. LEVELS OF ORGANIZATION AND MEDICAL SERVICES
IN CHINA'S RURAL AREAS

Organizational level	Population range	Medical facilities and personnel
Province or autonomous region (27 in China)	About 1 million to 50 million	Provincial hospitals—subspecialists, Western and traditional doctors, bureau of public health
County (2000 in China)	Up to 1 million	County hospitals—specialists, Western and traditional doctors
Commune (27 000 in China)	Up to 60 000	Commune hospitals or clinics—Western and traditional doctors, assistant doctors, nurses
Production brigade (5–20 per commune)	500–3000	Brigade health stations—barefoot doctors, health aides
Production team (10–30 per brigade)	50–300	Barefoot doctors, health aides

doctors, though from somewhat more elaborate health stations. The stations are generally furnished with an examination table, a desk and a few chairs, a medicine cabinet stocked with both traditional and Western medicine and an acupuncture chart hanging on the wall. The health care provided includes immunizations, health education, and the treatment of minor illness. Midwives also work from the brigade health stations; they perform normal deliveries in the mother's home and deal with birth control.

Many large communes have their own hospital facilities to which patients are referred from the production brigade health stations. In the 10 counties that comprise the Shanghai municipality, for example, there are 212 commune hospitals (at least one for every commune), with an average of 30 beds each.

Each county in China has a general hospital, which is usually located in the county town and serves the people of the immediate area as well as patients referred from the commune hospitals. To take an example, the hospital of Shunyi County, a part of Peking municipality north-east of the city proper, has a staff of 104 men and 114 women to run its ambulatory and inpatient services for the 450 000 members of the county's communes. Of this staff, 143 are medical workers—48 doctors (which probably includes "assistant doctors"), 63 nurses, and 32 pharmacists and technicians. In addition to this hospital, seven commune hospitals and 12 commune clinics provide medical care in the county. In all, 676 medical workers (excluding barefoot doctors and health aides) serve Shunyi County: 312 doctors, 65 nurses, and 299 pharmacists and technicians.

Medical care in the cities

Although 80% of China's population live in the rural areas, there are still about 150 million people in its cities, so that it also has one of the world's largest urban populations. The cities of China are densely crowded. The largest, Shanghai, has a population of about 6 million people living in the 140 km^2 of the city proper who, with the 5 million in the surrounding rural areas, make up Shanghai Municipality (7). The city proper thus has a population density of over 42 800 per km^2, about twice that of Manhattan Island in the USA and 10 times that of Singapore (2.2 million people in 585 km^2).

Since the Cultural Revolution, cities have been governed by revolutionary committees, which are formal government bodies. Their health services are coordinated by the local bureau of public health, which has responsibility not only for almost all service units and health care personnel in the city but also for educational institutions for non-physician health care personnel as well. Each city differs somewhat in the organization of its health services, so that generalizations are difficult.

Three cities and their supporting countryside areas have been removed from the jurisdiction of the provinces in which they are situated and placed directly under the central government as independent municipalities. The largest of these is Shanghai ; the others are Tientsin, with a population of 4 million, and Peking.

The Shanghai Bureau of Public Health may serve as an example of the functioning of municipal public health administration in China and its relationship with other community services. There are six departments in the Bureau : (1) curative medicine, pharmacy, hygiene, and public health, with jurisdiction over hospitals, maternal and child health, middle medical schools, occupational hygiene, communicable disease, pharmacies, and barefoot doctors : (2) medical research ; (3) emergency medical care ; (4) administration ; (5) finance ; and (6) personnel.

The Municipal Public Health Station, operated by the Department of Curative Medicine, Pharmacy, Hygiene, and Public Health, employs 300–400 staff, most of whom are assigned to district and county stations. They are responsible for epidemiology, sanitation, school health, and nutrition. There is also a Municipal Occupational Health Station with 200 inpatient beds, and a station in each district to supervise BCG vaccinations against tuberculosis. Each district has a dental station, often at the district hospital. There are mental health stations in each district as well as in a few counties. The Bureau is also responsible for maintaining statistics on Shanghai's health status.

Table 2 gives an outline of city health services in China. The next level of organization below the municipal level is the " district ", which is also governed by a revolutionary committee. Hangchow, a city of 700 000 people,

TABLE 2 LEVELS OF ORGANIZATION AND MEDICAL SERVICES
IN CHINA'S URBAN AREAS

Organizational level	Size of population	Medical facilities and personnel
Municipality	From less than 100 000 to 11 million (Shanghai, of which about 6 million would be considered urban)	Specialized and teaching hospitals—sub-specialists, bureau of public health
District	From less than 100 000 to 900 000 (a district in Shanghai)	District hospitals—specialists, epidemic prevention centres
Neighbourhoods (also called " streets " or " urban communes ")	40 000–70 000	Neighbourhood hospitals or clinics—Western-type doctors, traditional doctors, assistant doctors, nurses, midwives
Residents' committees (also called " lanes ")	1000–8000	Residents' committee or lane health stations—red medical workers with periodic visits by doctors
Group	50–150	

is divided into four districts; the city proper of Peking into nine districts; and the city proper of Shanghai into 10 districts. Districts are subdivided into " streets " or " neighbourhoods ", which are the lowest level of formal governmental organization in the city. The population of these neighbourhoods varies from approximately 40 000 to 70 000.

The neighbourhood is governed by a committee of representatives of the people in the area, cadres and, in diminishing numbers since the Cultural Revolution, members of the People's Liberation Army. The committee's responsibilities include the administration of local factories, primary schools and kindergartens, the neighbourhood hospital or health centre, repair services, and a housing department, and the organization and supervision of " residents' " or " lane " committees.

The smallest unit in the urban areas is usually the " lane " (or " residents' committee ") with 1000–8000 people. Some lanes are further divided into groups—for example, the residents of a single large apartment building—headed by a group or deputy group leader. The lane is governed by a committee chosen by, and from among, the " mass " living in the lane. The residents' committees are " mass organizations " rather than formal governmental bodies and do not usually have the components of the revolutionary committees; the elderly play a key role in their organization and administration (8).

In Peking city proper, each of the nine districts has a population of about 400 000. Among the services provided at the district level are hospitals, sanitation facilities, middle schools (roughly equivalent to junior and senior high schools), and " prevention stations " for illnesses such as tuberculosis and mental disorders.

Within each district are " neighbourhoods " of approximately 50 000 people. The West District of Peking has nine neighbourhoods, of which Fengsheng neighbourhood, with a population of 53 000, is one ; within this neighbourhood's jurisdiction are six factories, eight shops, 10 primary schools, four kindergartens, and a neighbourhood hospital (8).

The people of Fengsheng are grouped into 25 residents' committees, each of about 2000 people, which usually provide a health station and other social services. Within each committee are organized " groups " of 50–150 retired people and housewives (workers belong to groups at their place of work), led by a group leader and deputy group leader, who do what might be called social or welfare work.

The residents' committee health station is near the residents' homes and its major functions are preventive work, health education, birth control and the treatment of minor illnesses. The health workers at the residents' committee level are local housewives, who are called " red medical workers ". Health care is also given in factories, either by worker doctors or by fully trained physicians. Most factories have a central clinic as well as health stations in individual workshops ; often there is a factory hospital with beds for short-term stays.

The back-up institution for the residents' committees and the factory health stations is the neighbourhood hospital (which often has no beds and might be called a clinic in English). Neighbourhood hospitals are generally staffed by physicians fully trained in both traditional and Western medicine, and by middle medical workers (nurses, technicians and assistant doctors). They are the referral centres for the local health stations and in turn refer patients to district and specialty hospitals. For example, the Fengsheng Neighbourhood Hospital, which occupies two large courtyards, has seven departments—medicine, surgery, acupuncture, traditional bone medicine, gynaecology, dentistry, and tuberculosis—and four auxiliary units—pharmacy (including both traditional Chinese and Western drugs), laboratory, X-ray, and injections. The public health department serving the neighbourhood is located in the hospital ; patients requiring hospitalization are sent to the People's Hospital (the district hospital for the West District) several blocks from Fengsheng.

Although the equipment in the neighbourhood hospital is sparse and primitive, it seems adequate for the type of health work performed there. Facilities for simple laboratory tests and X-rays are available. In addition, the hospital acts as a centre for public health work in the neighbourhood.

Hospitals in China's cities range from these small neighbourhood hospitals to technologically sophisticated research and teaching hospitals. In Peking, for example, there are four research-oriented specialized hospitals under the aegis of the Academy of Medical Sciences ; 23 municipal hospitals,

10 of which have over 500 beds, under the jurisdiction of the Peking Bureau of Public Health ; and 20 district hospitals.

The theme of knowing by doing propounded in Mao Tse-tung's essay *On practice* (9) runs through essentially all aspects of Chinese life today. A peasant learns the difficulties of determining agricultural priorities by taking part in decision-making. The urban doctor learns about the life of the peasants by moving to the countryside for a while and labouring with them. The child learns what it is like to be a peasant or a worker by growing vegetables or doing jobs for a factory at home. According to this theory, the way to teach 800 million people the principles of health prevention and health care is to see that they are involved.

The mobilization of the masses has been China's main technique in accomplishing its feats of engineering : the construction of its canals and bridges, its large-scale irrigation projects, and the damming of its rivers. Mass mobilization has also been the key mechanism in its feats of human engineering. In health care this has meant the broadest involvement of people at every level of society in movements such as the Patriotic Health Campaign ; the recruitment of selected groups of people such as barefoot doctors from the population they are to serve ; and the mobilization of the individual to " fight against his own disease ". Individual concern with health reflects the Chinese belief in *tzu-li keng-sheng* or self-reliance, more accurately translated as " regeneration through one's own efforts "—a virtue as honoured today as its obverse, mutual help.

In the early 1950s, in accordance with the fourth of the main health principles—" health work should be combined with the mass movement "— the Patriotic Health Campaign was launched. The primary goal of the mass movement at that time was the elimination of mosquitos, flies, rats and sparrows (the sparrows were soon replaced on the list by bedbugs), and the people were mobilized to exterminate these pests under the guidance of health personnel. The Patriotic Health Campaign has been maintained and expanded to include the sanitary aspects of food, water, and the environment.

Health propaganda plays a crucial role in the participation of the community in health problems. Great attention is paid to educating the population on the importance of immunizations, the handling of infectious diseases, and the need for planned births.

The classic example of the use of mass organization in health has been the campaign against schistosomiasis. According to Horn (*10*) this campaign was based on the concept of the " mass line "—" the conviction that the ordinary people possess great strength and wisdom and that when their initiative is given full play they can accomplish miracles ". Before the peasants were organized to fight against the snails, they were thoroughly educated in the nature of schistosomiasis by means of lectures, films, posters, and radio talks. They were then mobilized twice a year, in March and August, and, along with voluntary labour from the People's Liberation Army, students, teachers, and office workers, they drained the rivers and ditches, buried the banks of the rivers, and smoothed down the surface. The idea was not only to recruit the people to do the work but to mobilize their enthusiasm and initiative so that they would fight the disease (11).

The elimination of venereal disease in China provides another example of both the mobilization and education of the people and the use of indigenous health personnel. In the early 1950s checklists of symptoms were posted in every store and community centre throughout the country, and anyone with any of the symptoms was urged to undergo a blood test and be treated. Neighbourhood pressure was brought to bear on those who ignored symptoms or had a history of promiscuity. Where the concentration of the disease was great, specially trained individuals made door-to-door visits to carry out examinations and blood tests. Prostitutes were identified and given suitable alternative work, if necessary by moving equipment, such as sewing machines, into the brothels and turning them into factories. Thus prostitution was outlawed. Neighbourhood committees had, and continue to have, the authority to eliminate prostitution and promiscuity (12, 13).

In health, as in other fields according to the Chinese brand of socialism, there are no passive bystanders. Each person is expected to participate wholeheartedly in community public health measures, the organization of medical care, and the conduct of all aspects of his or her personal life, including health. It is a country of mass and individual participation, of mass and individual responsibility. According to one observer (14), China views the role of the people thus :

> "To gain knowledge, people must be awakened from their half slumber, encouraged to mobilize themselves and to take conscious action to elevate and liberate themselves. When they actively participate in decision-making, when they take an interest in state affairs, when they dare to do new things, when they become good at presenting facts and reasoning things out, when they criticize and test and experiment scientifically, having discarded myths and superstitions, when they are aroused—then the socialist initiative latent in the masses will burst out with volcanic force".

Health manpower

There is no clear gradation from one level of health worker to another in China. Job assignments are based much more on demonstrated skills than on the possession of a specific degree or other credential or even the amount of previous education or experience. Nonetheless it is possible to divide China's health workers into rough categories :

Full-time workers :

    Higher medical workers :
        Doctors of Western medicine
        Stomatologists
        Pharmacologists

Doctors of Chinese medicine

Middle medical workers :
    Assistant doctors
    Nurses
    Midwives
    Pharmacists
    Technicians

Part-time workers :
    Barefoot doctors
    Worker doctors
    Red medical workers

Spare-time workers :
    Health aides

The education of doctors of Western medicine has undergone profound changes in recent years. Students now often leave school after completion of junior middle school, at about 16 years of age, to work for at least two years, and more likely three years, in a commune or factory. At the end of that time, if they are chosen by their fellow workers, they are admitted to universities, professional schools or technical schools. The criteria by which they are chosen include not only their intellectual accomplishments, but also the attitudes and principles they have expressed and lived by during their period of work. It is now said to be a person's " politics " and his " attitude toward the people " rather than how brilliant he is that determine whether he will be a good doctor or other kind of professional. Since 1971 some senior middle school graduates have also been admitted to medical school.

Not only were curricula generally shortened in the wake of the Cultural Revolution, but the practical content was markedly increased while the share of theory fell. Also, periods of direct work were included in all programmes. Thus a student studying physics now spends some of his time in factories learning how physics can be helpful in production and a student of biology spends time in the communes learning how biology can assist agriculture. The post-Cultural Revolution curriculum is said to " eliminate the irrelevant and the redundant " by combining the theoretical with the practical and by using the " three-in-one " principle of : teachers teach students ; students teach teachers ; and students teach students. New methods of teaching are being tried. In contrast to the past, students are encouraged to question what they are taught and to participate much more in the educational process.

Since the Cultural Revolution, considerable emphasis has been placed in all medical schools on teaching traditional medicine. In some cities, such as Nanking, the former traditional medical college has been combined with a Western-type medical college ; in others, such as Kwangchow and

Peking, the two types of college have informal links, and some graduates of Western medical colleges may attend traditional colleges for further work after graduation.

Middle medical workers are trained in middle medical schools. Before the Cultural Revolution the training lasted about three years. Since then, the training of assistant doctors is said not to have resumed at all and the training of nurses and other middle medical workers, which has started again in the past three years, has been shortened to about two years. Like all medical workers in China, they are given training in both Western-type and traditional Chinese medicine.

The part-time health workers—barefoot doctors, worker doctors, and red medical workers—are not thought of primarily as health workers at all; they are counted in the Chinese statistics—and apparently think of themselves—as primarily agricultural workers (barefoot doctors), production workers (worker doctors), or housewives or retired people (red medical workers). These part-time health workers (a) remain an integral part of the group they serve and (b) are part of a highly structured system that, while varying from place to place, seems usually to provide for adequate supervision, demand accountability, and permit appropriate referral.

Just as much of the work of the part-time health workers seems to vary from place to place in China, so too does their education. For the barefoot doctor the most frequent pattern appears to be a three-month period of formal training, either in the county hospital or in the commune hospital, fairly evenly divided between theoretical and practical work. The three-month training is followed by a variable period of on-the-job experience under supervision. As seems to be common in present-day China, continuing training either on the job or in further short courses enables workers to upgrade their skills. In practice, preference for entry to medical college goes to the barefoot doctors and other health workers because they are often the ones chosen by their fellow workers as most suitable for such training.

Conclusions

Faced with massive problems and extremely limited resources, China has over the course of 25 years created a society—and within that society a health care system—that has acted vigorously to meet the people's basic needs (15). While areas of very low population density clearly have less coverage than areas of high density, China has made great efforts to see that its still limited resources are distributed as equitably as possible. This is done, however, within the context of local self-reliance and initiative. The communes, which are the economic and political units of the rural areas, are responsible for health services for their members. They fulfil these responsibilities in part with the help of mobile medical teams and other health workers on rotation from the cities and some county or provincial training facilities, but for the most part with their own resources. Thus the coverage is still somewhat uneven, depending in part on the resources of the commune, but is much more equitable than in the past.

Precise figures for the use of health services are not available, but it seems clear that, following China's great efforts to merge traditional and modern medicine, many rural people are more and more willing to avail themselves of the combined system. The apparently highly successful efforts to stimulate mass participation in sanitation and other health movements seem also to encourage the use of therapeutic facilities.

The cost of health services in China appears quite low, although again exact figures are not available. Economy is attained by a combination of low-cost local facilities, the use of traditional techniques and medicines, modest salary levels for health workers, and an incentive system increasingly based on social motivation rather than economic rewards. While there is still often a direct charge to the patient at the time of service, it is low enough to be little or no barrier to access : most of the cost of health services is borne by regular family payments under cooperative schemes or by contributions from factory or commune income. At higher levels of specialization much of the cost is borne by the appropriate government agency.

Perhaps the most difficult assessment in this analysis is the degree to which China's experience is applicable to other developing countries. It is often said that because China's social, economic, political and cultural circumstances differ so markedly from those of other countries, there is little in the Chinese experience that can be directly transferred. While this may be true—and Chinese representatives have themselves frequently stated that each country must find solutions to its problems based on its own special circumstances—there are basic principles that may indeed be relevant to other societies. These include the emphasis on local self-reliance, on brief training and structured part-time use of locally recruited and locally trained people, on the combination of modern and traditional medicine, and on preventive medicine. Perhaps even more important—if difficult to implement—are the beliefs that fundamental changes in health and health care may require fundamental changes in the social structure in which they are embedded, that equitable distribution of resources must be a basic goal of society, and that the opportunity to be of service should be a prime motivating force in health work as in other human services. But surely the greatest lesson that China offers is that it can be done—that a nation can within one generation move from a starving, sickness-riddled, illiterate, élitist semi-feudal society to a vigorous, healthy, productive, highly literate, mass participation society. If China can accomplish it, other nations can too.

REFERENCES

1. First Five-Year Plan for Development of the National Economy of the People's Republic of China in 1953–1957, Peking, Foreign Language Press, 1956, pp. 199–200.

2. ORLEANS, L. A. Medical education and manpower in communist China. In: C. T. Hu, ed. *Aspects of Chinese education*, New York, Teachers College Press, Colombia University, 1969.

3. CHANG TZE-K'UAN. The development of hospital services in China. *Chinese Medical Journal*, **84** : 412–416 (1965).

4. SHABAD, T. *China's changing map*, rev. ed. New York, Praeger, 1972.

5. THOMSON, J. C., Jr. *While China faced West*, Boston, Mass., Harvard University Press, 1971.

6. HINTON, W. *Fanshen*, New York, Vintage Books, 1966.

7. LAMM, S. H. & SIDEL, V. W. Analysis of preliminary public health data for Shanghai, 1972. In: SIDEL, V.W. & SIDEL, R. *Serve the people : Observations on medicine in the People's Republic of China*, Boston, Mass., Beacon Press, 1974, pp. 238-166.

8. SIDEL, R. *Families of Fengsheng : Urban life in China*, New York, Penguin, 1974.

9. MAO TSE-TUNG. On practice. In: *Four Essays on philosophy*, Peking, Foreign Language Press, 1966, p. 8.

10. HORN, J. S. *Away with all pests ... An English surgeon in People's China*, New York, Monthly Review Press, 1971, p. 126.

11. *Ibid.*, p. 96.

12. SNOW, E. *Red China today*, New York, Vintage Books, 1970, pp. 261–269.

13. HATEM, G. With Mao Tse-tung's thought as the compass for action in the control of venereal disease in China. *China's Medicine*, 1 October 1966, pp. 52–67.

14. GURLEY, J. G. Capitalist and Maoist economic development. In: FREEDMAN, E. & SELDEN, M., ed. *America's Asia*, New York, Vintage Books, 1971, p. 336.

15. SIDEL, V.W. & SIDEL, R. *Serve the people: Observations on medicine in the People's Republic of China*, Boston, Mass., Beacon Press, 1974.

Cuba's health care system [a]

Background

Cuba is an island with an estimated population of 9 170 000 (1972). The average population density is 77.1 persons per km². The climate is subtropical.

Agriculture is the most important economic activity. The world's biggest producer of sugar, Cuba is now diversifying its products, with particular attention to increasing the output of animal protein to cover the population's needs. Industry is also being developed.

The JUCEPLAN (Junta Central de Planificación) is the government unit responsible for overall planning.

---

[a] Visit made and case study prepared by Dr S. Gomez (WHO), Dr E. Liisberg (WHO), Mr A. Robles (UNICEF), and Dr I. Tabibzadeh (WHO).

The situation up to 1959

Until the revolution in 1959 a considerable part of Cuba's population, especially in rural areas, had no access to any form of health services. The Government had a badly organized and inadequate service, mainly in towns. Private pharmacies, *curanderos* (" spiritualist " and " religious " healers) and traditional birth attendants (*comadronas empíricas*) served a considerable number of the population. Social insurance groupings (*mutualistas*) covered selected groups of industrial workers. The medical school in Havana turned out 300–400 doctors a year, most of whom took up private practice in the capital or other big towns, or emigrated. Private practice was subject to practically no control and varied widely in quality. There was no planned development of health services.

The prerevolutionary situation can be summarized as follows :

1. Absence of a national health system, of elementary coordination of existing services, and of vertical programmes to solve priority problems.

2. Insufficient services, the population being left to its own resources for medical attention, which for many people was unobtainable under those circumstances.

3. The low quality of state services compared with private services, which were generally very costly.

4. Predominantly curative services, and a virtual absence of preventive medicine.

5. Divorce between the teaching of medicine and social needs, doctors being trained for private curative practice.

The conceptual basis for Cuba's present approach

Cuba's experience in the health field derives from the transformation of its socioeconomic political structure in the period following the revolution in 1959. The priority given to and the changes made in health services at that time were a political decision based on the needs of the population as seen by the political leadership, which included a number of physicians. Health, education, and means of communication continue to have the highest socioeconomic development priority in Cuba and receive a considerable portion of the Government's budget and attention. Health care is considered a human right and an excellent political investment. Health services are free and run by the State. Equal distribution of services is a political dictum and is gradually being achieved. The health services are based on the following four basic principles :

— The health of the population is a government responsibility.

— Health services should be available to all the population.

— The community should participate actively in health work.

— Preventive and curative health services should be integrated.

Planning is pragmatic and based on the scientific use of epidemiological data and the experience of other countries.

WHO's policies are being followed with regard to regionalization, the use of auxiliaries, planning and programming, the eradication of specific diseases, maternal and child health, and other elements of health care.

Health action taken

At the beginning of 1960, the Government decided that the State should be responsible for health. Full responsibility was given to the Ministry of Health for the development of health services, the setting of norms and the implementation of policy.

In the period 1960-61, it was decided to require all new medical graduates to serve for six months in rural areas. They were sent to these areas to develop health services with whatever means were available, and to select persons who could be trained as auxiliaries.

The approach to the development of the health services was and is pragmatic and gradual. Private practice still continues (350 physicians), and the last *mutualista* (private group insurance) hospital was absorbed in 1970; during its last years it was run by the Ministry of Health as a *mutualista* hospital serving only the original members.

In 1961 a national medical meeting, attended by 2000 physicians (out of 5000 in Cuba), was held in Havana to explain to the medical profession the principles decided upon for the future development of the Cuban health services—full state responsibility, availability of services to all the population, community participation, and integrated services. Improved service conditions and possibilities for advanced training were also announced.

WHO's basic principles for the organization and development of health services were taken into account in the development of the services, and the implementation was gradual and pragmatic. In 1961-62 a series of specific vertical programmes was established (reduction of gastroenteritis, tuberculosis, polio and malaria, immunization against diphtheria, pertussis and tetanus, reduction of maternal mortality). To support the vertical programmes, health education teams were created to help prepare the community.

In October 1962 the country was organized into districts responsible for all activities. The district medical officer was placed in full charge of all the health services in the district, including private practice. With some modifications, the districts corresponded to the present regions, which were eventually found to be too big to handle as units and were divided into areas and sectors. The health system is now fully regionalized with well defined functions at every level and centralization of inpatient (specialist) care and decentralization of outpatient (primary) care.

In order to develop a well integrated health programme for rural areas, a pilot scheme was set up, with a health team responsible for 8 fields : integrated care for children ; integrated care for women ; integrated care for adults ; communicable diseases ; environmental sanitation ; food hygiene ; occupational health ; and dentistry. After six months the pilot study was showing successful results. Subsequently, health centres with the same programme were gradually established all over the country, with the emphasis on underdeveloped areas. In rural areas the centres, with 10–30 beds, are called rural hospitals ; in towns they are called polyclinics. In 1965 the hospitals were regionalized under great difficulties because of their very uneven distribution (for example, in Havana 90% of all hospital beds were in one area). A general plan for hospital construction, with priority to areas without services, was prepared in coordination with the plans of the political and other authorities, and a final decision on the overall plans were made by the central Government.

In 1963 a small group of gynaecologists-obstetricians drew up a set of norms for the diagnosis and treatment of certain specific conditions related to pregnancy (toxaemia, rupture of the uterus, etc.). The norms were based on specialist knowledge at that time. National norms for performance and techniques have since been developed over the years by task forces in many fields (paediatrics, obstetrics/gynaecology, surgery, statistics and others). They are based on a consensus of health workers in the particular field and on generally accepted medical knowledge. The norms, which are intended as a guide and not a straightjacket (la norma no es la horma), are distributed all over the country and are used in basic and in-service training, supervisory work, and the preparation of programmes and plans.

Training courses for different types of health staff were organized. The Ministry of Health was reorganized to deal with its extended and changing responsibilities, and norms were developed for different kinds of health staff and different specialties. It was decided not to utilize the existing traditional midwives and witch-doctors (curanderos). The witch-doctors were forbidden to practise, while the traditional midwives were gradually absorbed into the health services system, mostly as ancillary staff.

At the start of the 1960s most trained health workers were auxiliaries. At present the great majority of trained personnel are of the middle level. Thirty-four nurses' training schools run by the Ministry of Health are now producing nurses with three years' training, starting with tenth-grade students. The nurses' schools are scattered in all the provinces so as to favour all areas equally and to allow students to work in their home districts when they qualify. Middle-level technicians receive two-three years of training in provincial or national schools. More than 20 types of technicians are trained, including technicians for the maintenance of equipment and buildings. Auxiliaries in both the nursing and the technical fields are also trained in large numbers. The needs in the different fields are carefully studied and training programmes are established accordingly. Staff functions are well defined and training (including social motivation) is adapted to the jobs to be performed.

The number of health staff is increasing rapidly because of expanding training programmes and health worker/population ratios are improving; in 1971 there were 9.2 auxiliary nurses, 5.5 professional nurses and about 10 physicians per 10 000 inhabitants.

Supervision and control

Regular technical and administrative supervision and control operate from the top to the bottom of the organization in a continuous and systematic way. There are no special supervisory teams; every person from the central, provincial and regional level supervises the part of the organization below him, including the clinicians who belong to the normative groups. The deputy ministers go to a different province once a month to look at the programmes in their charge. This ensures that each province is scrutinized at least once a year. These visits cover not only the provincial headquarters but district and area establishments as well.

Besides this administrative and technical control, the government party and the mass organizations play an active role in seeing that the political directions given by the hierarchy are followed.

The supervisor gives actual assistance to those supervised in difficult tasks such as programming and evaluation; teaching is considered a very important part of supervision and is effectively carried out.

Teamwork

The concept of teamwork goes beyond the classical coordination of activities of the local group for the direct delivery of services to the population. Each health worker at every level has the same philosophy and a very clear understanding of what his responsibility is in the accomplishment of the goals. Unified groups have been created that cross the boundaries of age, occupational status, level of training and disciplines.

The five most important factors in the *esprit de corps* pervading the health teams seem to be:

1. All health staff belong to the same union, which gives them a common sense of interest and responsibility and does away with factionalism in the approach to problems.

2. Regular meetings are held with all the staff at which all are expected to give their opinion and participate.

3. Clearly defined duties and responsibilities and a well defined system of interrelationships are established.

4. Indirect (and direct) pressure is exerted from the community, the mass organizations and the party, through the established system of participation by the different groups at all levels, for the creation of a team approach geared towards solving the community's problems.

5. All levels and units take part in the planning of activities; this imparts a stronger sense of participation in the health system and possibly results in a more realistic planning of its activities.

On the basis of the experience gained, a more structured programming process with more specific objectives and targets has been developed. Since 1963 emphasis has also been put on developing an information system to be used in defining problems and monitoring progress.

Environmental sanitation

There seems to be an imbalance between environmental sanitation and medical care, especially in the rural areas. For example, the rapid decline in mortality due to diarrhoeal diseases (from 68 deaths per 100 000 inhabitants in 1962 to approximately 15 in 1972) has not been accompanied by a similar decline in morbidity. In fact, the decline in mortality has been achieved by an intensive programme of health education, early detection of cases and early hospitalization. This is linked with the general policy of bringing the scattered rural population together into aggregations around the production programmes. All new rural housing projects fulfil all the sanitation requirements in relation to water supply, sewage disposal, and vector and rat control.

In 1974, a project was under study at central government level to meet sanitation needs in the period 1976-1980.

Population involvement and mass mobilization

The whole population is enrolled in the fight against disease. A massive channelling of women into socially useful work has made a great contribution in this respect. At the local level, whether the rural hospital or the polyclinic, people's health commissions are active. These commissions are presided over by the physician-director of the health institution and each of the mass or community organizations—e.g., Committees for the Defence of the Revolution, the Federation of Cuban Women, and the labour unions—is represented. In the rural areas a member of the National Association of Small Farmers, which belongs to the private sector, also participates. The team is completed by a party representative. The commissions meet regularly and a great diversity of problems is discussed, such as school-children's vaccination and the hygiene of local milk production.

The Committees for the Defence of the Revolution alone group together over 3.5 million adults. Their primary level of organization corresponds to city blocks in the urban areas and to large farms in the rural areas. In the field of public health their first task, in conjunction with the health services, was immunization of the whole population. Other important activities were the removal of animals from near houses and the elimination of rubbish to avoid the proliferation of flies and other disease carriers. The use of such an organization makes it possible to vaccinate one and a half million children with oral poliomyelitis vaccine in a few hours at almost no expense. The free availability of all mass media, including radio, press, and television, makes it easy to approach the people. The reasons for each health activity are explained. Each member of every health team is trained to adopt a community approach as a health educator or orientation-giver. New physicians are trained in contact with the community from their first year of study.

Costs

No absolute figures are available for expenditure on health, but 50% or more of the government budget is allocated to health and education.

Leprosy and tuberculosis control, and selected health indicators

Ninety-nine per cent of leprosy patients and 85.4% (1972) of contacts are regularly supervised. More than 90% of the population has been covered by the programme for the diagnosis and treatment of tuberculosis. BCG vaccinations are administered to about 95% of the newborn and repeat vaccinations are given to all children in primary schools.

The health indicators tabulated below show some of the results achieved by Cuba's present health system (figures supplied by the Government):

Mortality rates (per 1000)

Crude death rate	6.5	(1958)	5.8	(1973)
Infant mortality rate	33.0	(1958)	27.0	(1973)
Mortality rate, age 1–4 years	2.6	(1958)	1.2	(1970)
Maternal mortality rate	1.2	(1962)	0.6	(1972)
Stillbirths	25.0	(1962)	13.0	(1972)

Disease-specific mortality rates (per 100 000)

Gastroenteritis	42.5	(1957)	18.4	(1970)
Tuberculosis	19.6	(1962)	7.3	(1970)
Typhoid	0.2	(1968)	0.0	(1971)
Poliomyelitis	32	cases (1960)	no cases since 1972	
Malaria	eradicated			

Morbidity rates (per 100 000)

Poliomyelitis	eradicated (342 cases reported in 1961)		
Whooping cough	15.6	(1967–1969)	7.2 (1970–1972)
Tetanus	4.3	(1967–1969)	2.3 (1970–1972)
Tetanus neonatorum	49.0	(1959)	0.0 (1970)—1 case
Diphtheria	2.6	(1967–1969)	0.0 (1971–1973)
Tuberculosis	41.0	(1968)	17.8 (1971)

Conclusions

Cuba has a health service system accessible and available to practically 100% of the population, with a referral system ensuring the appropriate level of care for each patient. Preventive, curative and rehabilitation services are well planned and integrated and show excellent results in terms of service indicators and mortality and morbidity data.

Certain factors have helped to make the Cuban health services efficient, such as extremely high motivation of the health services, complete literacy, a high proportion of doctors and other health professional staff, good transport facilities, mass mobilization and full participation of the people.

United Republic of Tanzania : An innovative approach to the development of health services[a]

General situation

The United Republic of Tanzania's approach to meeting the health needs of the majority of its population must be considered in the light of the constraints imposed by its lack of financial resources and manpower—it is one of the 25 countries with the lowest per capita gross national product in the world—and also of its colonial past, which left it with a minimal health infrastructure to build upon following independence.

Tanzania has a land mass of approximately 1 million km². Much of the country is dry ; large areas are covered by scrub and grassland, except in the region surrounding Mount Kilimanjaro where rainfall is good. In 1972, the population was estimated at about 13.5 million. The birth rate was 47 per 1000 and the crude death rate estimated at 20 per 1000, giving a natural growth rate of 2.7% a year. As in most developing countries, the life expectancy at birth is very low (44 years). The infant mortality rate is 160–165 per 1000. The people are agropastoral, with 92.5% of the sparse population living in the rural areas.

Again as in most developing countries, reliable statistics about the disease pattern in Tanzania are not available. Most of the morbidity and

---

[a] Visit made and case study prepared by Dr V. Djukanovic (WHO), Dr E. Kalimo (WHO), and Dr I. M. Omari (UNICEF).

mortality results from communicable diseases of an endemo-epidemic nature (no less than 50 communicable diseases have been diagnosed). Nutritional diseases, complications following pregnancy and delivery, and chronic and degenerative diseases are also found. The causes of mortality have been ranked as follows : acute respiratory diseases, measles, enteritis and diarrhoea, malaria, nutritional diseases including malnutrition, and complications following pregnancy and delivery. In spite of the lack of complete data, this list clearly indicates the epidemiological priorities and health needs facing the Tanzanian health authorities.

In 1973, mainland Tanzania had 128 hospitals with 18 700 beds, or one hospital bed per 720 inhabitants. There were 105 rural health centres, 1500 rural dispensaries, and some 1500 health posts at village level. Each rural health centre was then intended to provide health services for 187 000 inhabitants and each dispensary covered about 9300 people. However, the distribution of services varies from region to region. At the end of 1972 there was one physician per 28 000 population, with a correspondingly low ratio of other health professionals and auxiliaries ; these figures reflect the overall shortage of health manpower.

National policy for socioeconomic development

Given the prevailing economic, social and technological context of Tanzania, there was a clear need for a national will to bring about a chance. This will was enunciated in the 1967 Arusha Declaration, which forms the basis of Tanzania's current health policy. Health was to be viewed within the framework of the national socioeconomic plan, with the main emphasis on rural development. The Arusha Declaration calls for :

— Overall rural development.

— Government mobilization of all resources for the elimination of poverty, ignorance and disease.

— Active participation by the Government in the formation and maintenance of cooperative organizations.

— A contribution from the people (self-reliance) as an instrument for self-liberation and social development.

— People, land, good policies and good leadership as prerequisites of development.

It was decided to decentralize the planning machinery so that the people themselves could participate in the formulation of plans that would change their socioeconomic status. Hence planning committees were established at each village, ward and district level, with the National Ministry of Economic Planning setting the broad outlines of national planning priorities and strategy. However, significant government efforts only began in 1972/73, when about 70% of the budget was devoted to rural development. International organizations and other donor agencies have played a part in implementing the Government's objective of rural development, but " cooperation and not poisoned aid " remains the national theme.

The national socioeconomic plan aims at developing an integrated basic health infrastructure that will be acceptable and accessible to most of the population within Tanzania's social, economic and cultural framework, at the lowest possible cost. Other components of development in rural areas to be given prominence include the provision of safe water and free primary education for all. Health services plans have been formulated at different levels and coordinated with national development plans, in which the promotion and restoration of the health of the population are used as guiding principles.

In accordance with the Arusha Declaration, self-reliance was stressed. Local contributions in cash and kind were encouraged, giving the population an important role in the establishment of social services and necessary facilities. Mass mobilization was used as a political tool to enhance the social consciousness of the people, who were encouraged to take responsibility for meeting their socioeconomic needs as far as possible. Mass mobilization has also been applied in health educational activities, with emphasis on health promotion, the prevention of disease, and curative care.

To make it easier to provide essential social services, people in rural areas were encouraged to regroup in larger villages called Ujamaa villages. This regroupment scheme tends to minimize the worst problems of planning for sparsely populated communities, achieving a wider coverage of the population more easily. To make self-reliance a reality, village health posts and dispensaries are constructed by the villagers themselves, the Government providing the necessary materials, equipment, and services not obtainable locally. The villagers also participate in the construction of their water supply system and are encouraged to build their own pit latrines and rubbish dumps.

Manpower development and resources

Because of the shortage of manpower and resources in relation to the growing health demands from the rapidly increasing population, a departure from the traditional ways of providing health manpower had to be made. Tanzania's system now uses specially trained development workers at village level. These workers are given special courses in health improvement, especially in preventive medicine, which enables them to guide rural development with the required emphasis on health. They also help to stimulate the community to recognize their main health problems and jointly to work out solutions, using locally available resources.

Following the national principle of decentralization and mass mobilization, the health services organization was decentralized in July 1972, in an attempt to put most of the decision-making machinery in the hands of the people themselves in the regions, districts, and villages.

In each region there is a regional medical officer, who is a member of the regional development committee. He is at the same time the director of the regional hospital and coordinator for the implementation of health policy in his region. At the district level there is a district medical officer, who has the same functions in his district. Rural areas have health centres, dispensaries and, at the village level, village health posts.

The rural health centres and dispensaries are intended to provide comprehensive health services for the rural communities. However, the imbalance between curative and preventive activities still looms large, even in rural areas. The main aim of the development of rural health manpower in Tanzania is to staff the rural health services with primary health workers. Four main categories are involved : medical assistants, rural medical aides, maternal and child health aides, and health auxiliaries. Activities at each rural health centre and dispensary can be broadly divided into three : diagnosis and treatment, maternal and child health work, and environmental health work. The training of staff for these activities in rural areas is part of the rural development programme. The use of primary health workers in rural areas contributes to the equitable distribution of scarce health resources, leading to wider coverage of the population and better utilization of available health services at minimum cost.

A village medical helper in an Ujamaa village is supported by his village, with a rural health centre providing technical supervision and the central Government supplying equipment and drugs. His training in health is a practical first-aid course, lasting three to six months, at a health centre or at the district hospital. The aim is to repeat the courses periodically.

The maternal and child health aide, formerly the village midwife, is responsible for maternal and child welfare, including family planning and nutrition education. It is intended that the aide should work in two places, at the dispensary and at the rural health centre. She will be the only maternal and child health worker at the dispensary level but, more often than not, she is likely to be an assistant to a trained nurse at the health centre level.

Health auxiliaries have been specially trained and employed for environmental health in the rural areas for the past six years or so. They are employed at both health centres and dispensaries.

A rural medical aide has at least primary education and receives his medical training in a course lasting at least three years. Planners in Tanzania stress that the training of a rural medical aide should not consist of a watered-down programme for physicians. The syllabus is based on the requirements and goals of a dispensary and the aides' most common activities.

The most important institution in Tanzania's rural health services is the rural health centre. Since the medical assistant is trained to be in charge of such a centre, his is the most important category of rural health staff. With an educational background of at least 11 years of general schooling, the medical assistant is given three years of medical education comprising basic medical sciences, clinical medicine, and community medicine.

The assistant medical officer bears the title of doctor, is originally trained as a medical assistant, and then has at least four years' work experience followed by an 18-month training course. He performs functions somewhere between those of a medical assistant and a physician.

The philosophy of training doctors in Tanzania is to meet local needs and problems. In addition to performing clinical tasks, doctors must be health organizers and administrators of health teams. This implies that part of a doctor's training should take place in rural communities. In the medical faculty of the University of Dar es Salaam, community medicine is taught throughout the 200-week course of study and at least 22 weeks must be spent in communities doing field work.

The figures that follow illustrate the strategy and the action taken to achieve total coverage by rural health services. In 1971 there were 74 rural medical aides, in 1972 the number had increased to 578, and between 1973 and 1980 intensive training will be organized for peripheral primary health workers with an expected total output by 1980 of about 2500.

Medical assistants did not exist in 1961. In 1972 there were 335, and it is expected that by 1980 there will be more than 1500. The total number of assistant medical officers in 1961 was 22, in 1972 there were 140, and in 1980 it is expected that there will be about 400. Particular emphasis will be placed on the training of maternal and child health aides; the total expected by 1980 is more than 2000.

At the same time the number of health centres will be increased from 105 in 1973 to 300 by 1980, and the number of dispensaries from 1500 to 2300. The number of hospital beds will be increased only to maintain the same bed/population ratio.

Government health expenditure has risen from TSh 50 million [a] in the fiscal year 1961/62 to over four times that amount in 1973/74. The larger part of this increase occurred between 1971 and 1974. Although the absolute volume is small—about TSh 15 per person, plus an estimated additional TSh 3 per person on health in the private sector, giving a total of TSh 18 per person—Tanzania spends about 3% of its gross national product directly on health care (excluding water supply, sanitation, nutrition and other indirect but important determinants of health).

---

[a] 1 Tanzanian shilling = US $0.14 (1974).

Conclusion

In spite of the attractive and varied innovative features of Tanzania's health services, the health situation in the country in 1974 was far from ideal in terms of coverage and quality. Tanzania still has to face problems and difficulties that reflect its past history. Although its financial resources are modest, they are not the only constraint on the rapid development of health services; other factors are the lack of suitably trained health manpower and a sociocultural background that prevents the maximum usage of the existing system. However, rapid development in the health field and other socioeconomic developments in recent years suggest that the basic health needs of the majority of the population will be met during this decade.

Although the Tanzanian programme has to be understood in the context of the strong sociopolitical atmosphere prevailing in the country, the innovative characteristics of the approach could be adapted in tackling the pressing health problems of any developing country with similar health problems but with a different sociopolitical system. The approach is attractive in that it clearly demonstrates what can be done with minimum resources. What is needed is a strong national will, an objective examination of the health problems of the country, clear definition of targets, programmes and priorities in planning, and close adherence to a definite policy in the allocation of resources and the implementation of measures.

Venezuela : The "simplified medicine" programme [a]

Venezuela, with its 10 081 568 inhabitants at the 1971 census and an annual population growth rate of approximately 3.5% over the last 10 years, shows the trends and characteristics typical of developing societies

TABLE 3. SELECTED VITAL STATISTICS OF VENEZUELA
FOR 1950, 1960 AND 1970

	1950	1960	1970
Population (in millions)	5.0	7.4	9.8
Population aged 0–14 years (%)	42.6	44.8	47.1 [a]
Crude birth rate per 1000 population	42.8	44.0	41.0
Life expectancy at birth (years)	58.0	66.1	65.6 [b]
Crude death rate per 1000 population	10.9	7.5	7.0
Infant mortality per 1000 live births	79.7	55.2	48.2
Death at age 1–4 years per 1000 population	11.7	6.1	5.4
Proportionate undiagnosed mortality (%)	48.2	30.3	23.0

[a] 1971 census.
[b] For 1968.

[a] Visit made and case study prepared by Dr E. Liisberg (WHO), Mr A. Robles (UNICEF), Dr I. Tabibzadeh (WHO), and Dr F. Vargas Tentori (WHO).

with a high rate of growth and a preponderance of young people. The great changes in economic and social conditions over the past three decades have been reflected in levels of health. Tables 3 and 4 give an idea of the trends of certain health indicators and of the decrease in incidence of some communicable diseases.

TABLE 4. CASES OF SELECTED ACUTE DISEASES PER 100 000 POPULATION FOR THE NOTIFICATION AREA [a] OF VENEZUELA

Diseases	1950	1960	1970
Diphtheria	38.3	16.5	2.0
Typhoid fever	57.3	25.7	1.7
Malaria	80.0	25.0	10.5
Measles	342.2	517.0	496.6
Tetanus	26.8	22.9	5.1
Poliomyelitis	4.2	8.3	0.7
Smallpox	82.6	—	—
Murine typhus	6.7	0.4	—

[a] The part of Venezuela with a permanent medical service (including a physician). This contained an estimated 53.2% of the population in 1950, 60% in 1960, and 72.5% in 1970.

However, these data require further analysis. Venezuela, like many other developing countries, presents great contrasts between large urban concentrations of population (with the increasing problems of marginal areas as urbanization continues) and rural populations living in small villages or isolated *ranchos* with a rudimentary economy. Table 5 illustrates the variations of some health indices in different types of locality.

TABLE 5. MORTALITY INDICATORS IN FOUR POPULATION AGGREGATES, VENEZUELA, 1969

	Type of population aggregate			
	A	B	C	D
Crude death rate per 1000	6.1	8.1	8.4	8.0
Proportionate mortality by age (%):				
under 1 year	25.7	28.9	28.4	28.4
1–4 years	7.4	10.8	11.6	14.3
50 years and over	49.4	39.5	39.3	35.5
Proportionate undiagnosed mortality (%)	5.7	17.4	26.8	50.2

A: Population 40 000 and above.
B: Population 5000–39 999.
C: Population 1000–4999.
D: Population under 1000.

According to the 1971 census, of the 21 120 population centres in the country, there are 20 535 with 2500 or fewer persons in rural and intermediate areas, representing 27.26% of the total population. Thus, although urbanization has been rapid in Venezuela, the population is still very scattered and it is difficult to provide it with services, including basic medical care.

These considerations led a group of professionals in the Ministry of Health and Social Welfare to make an organized effort to establish a programme offering basic care for the scattered population, with due regard for the country's resources. The idea was to work out a simple, realistic, but practical approach to the problem. In 1961, at the Second Venezuelan Conference on Public Health, it was proposed to adapt experiments from other countries, particularly the USSR and certain African countries. It was obviously not feasible to place a doctor or other highly educated medical worker permanently in several thousand rural localities. There were already some 1300–1400 rural dispensaries, which were visited once a week or fortnight by a doctor from a town health centre to treat patients. In each dispensary an untrained girl was employed to help the doctor, do some cleaning and, if she could, apply dressings and give intramuscular injections.

The group of professionals studied the alternatives adopted in other countries in the light of local circumstances and existing facilities in Venezuela. As a result, it proposed that a new category of staff, called " health technicians ", should be created to diagnose and treat easily recognized diseases in a standard way and to be responsible for basic sanitation. The Ministry of Health gave the idea its backing, but the medical profession at first reacted unfavourably. The Venezuela Medical Federation invited the group to prepare a document explaining the experiment. This document, presented to the Federation in 1963, described the programme under the title " Simplified medicine " : medicine, to indicate that a comprehensive service, covering both preventive and curative aspects, would be provided ; and simplified, to indicate that it would consist of simple procedures of frontline medical care, but at the same time would have the necessary support from higher levels of the organized services. The Federation resolved to support the programme.

Simplified medicine as now established offers basic health care to the rural population through auxiliary health staff working within the health services, which provide continuous supervision, training and referral facilities. Each rural dispensary in the programme has an auxiliary health worker, who has to cover from 500 to a few thousand people, depending on how scattered the population is. The basic components of the care provided are as follows :

1. Promotion of health through elementary services for mothers and children, health education, and environmental sanitation.

2. Protection of health, mainly through immunization.

3. Restoration of health through first aid or simplified therapeutic action.

4. Registration of vital events.

64

5. Surveillance of certain diseases such as malaria and tuberculosis.

There are certain criteria for the selection of trainee auxiliaries :

— they must belong to the locality or be permanent residents ;
— they must be acceptable to local leaders ;
— they must be aged 18–40 years ;
— they must have had six years of primary schooling.

Most of the trainees are women, though male auxiliaries are preferred for the most remote or difficult areas. The programme for the training course follows an instruction manual, which is the auxiliary nurses' authority for their work. It gives explicit instructions on the type of preventive and curative medicine to be undertaken and on when and how to refer cases to a higher level. It authorizes treatment for recognizable common ailments such as diarrhoea in infants, and indicates how these are to be treated by diet and medicine that will not injure the patient. The auxiliaries are taught how to administer first aid for accidents while waiting for the doctor, and to educate local midwives and teach members of the families in their community how to protect children from birth to school age and beyond. They are also encouraged to cooperate with auxiliary personnel in other fields such as education, agriculture, and social welfare. The manual also explains, for example, how vaccination may be ineffective through faulty administration or a lack of facilities for preservation of the vaccine.

From the beginning it was decided that the auxiliaries' training should be essentially oriented to their future work. They are given the minimum of essential theoretical knowledge and concentrate on developing skills for :

1. Identifying diseases (or syndromes) that are easily recognizable and of relative frequency in the rural environment ;

2. Applying simple measures to promote, protect, and restore health, keeping to very clear guidelines in order to avoid abuses ;

3. Coordinating their efforts with the work of others involved in the progress of the community (teachers, home demonstrators, police, etc.).

The training courses are held in district health centres and never in a state capital, which might have an unsettling effect on the auxiliary nurse. The teaching staff consists of specially trained graduate nurses. The director of the district health centre exercises technical supervision and, together with other health staff from the district, gives lectures and arranges patient and group demonstrations. The teaching is essentially practical, with no theoretical teaching other than that contained in the manual. The students are not taught to deliver babies, but simply to supervise the local indigenous midwife and ensure a hygienic approach. The number of students on a training course, which lasts four months, usually does not exceed 12.

Supervision of the trained auxiliaries is provided through periodic visits (usually once a week or fortnight) by the doctor from the rural medical post or the health centre to which the dispensary is assigned, and visits by the regional nurses' supervisor. Experience in Venezuela has shown that for this job it is preferable to use a male graduate nurse, since he must travel a lot, spend nights in villages with little comfort, and stay as long as may be required for a satisfactory review of the auxiliary's work and for the correction of any defects, which might take several days. Because of the type of initial training received by the auxiliaries, it must be supplemented by in-service training, which is one of the objectives of supervision by the nurse. The supervisory visits by the nurse vary in frequency depending on circumstances, but an average of every three months is usual.

Most of the cost of health services in Venezuela is borne by the national and state governments. Some municipalities contribute, but in general their contribution is not substantial. One of the objectives of the simplified medicine programme in Venezuela is to encourage communities to participate more actively. Since health care is free, communities do not need to contribute to its financing. Nevertheless, there is some community participation, for instance in the cost of maintaining and running buildings and the construction and equipping of dispensaries.

Summary of results

Up to the end of 1973, 315 dispensaries in 12 states (out of 23 main political divisions) had been staffed by auxiliary health workers trained in simplified medicine. They cover a rural population of about 280 000 (the total rural population is 2.3 million). The programme has developed slowly and spread gradually from state to state. Among the 12 states involved in the simplified medicine programme, one or two have achieved a high coverage of the rural population.

The auxiliaries give the most essential vaccinations as a matter of routine, and watch for cases of tuberculosis and malaria. Pregnant women are followed up for any abnormalities and are referred to the rural doctor if necessary. Hospital delivery is encouraged, particularly for first babies. Local midwives meet periodically at the village dispensaries for discussions and to review the contents of their bags ; they are trained by the auxiliary nurses in hygienic delivery. Children are followed up regularly for vaccinations, weight control, supervision of feeding, etc. ; those with signs of malnutrition receive supplementary feeding. Pregnant women also receive supplementary food as well as iron tablets.

Elementary medical care is one of the major activities of the programme. The auxiliary gives treatment (including penicillin, sulfonamides, and other basic drugs) in cases he is able to diagnose (e.g., diarrhoea, dysentery, pneumonia). He must not go beyond this. Great use is made of referrals to the nearest health centre or rural doctor. No car or bicycles are assigned to dispensaries. Home visiting is carried out on foot.

Health education is given at the dispensary and through home visits, special mothers' classes, children's clubs and community meetings.

No serious attempts have been made to evaluate this programme from the viewpoint of coverage, utilization and cost/benefit. It would be difficult, if not impossible, to quantify the role of simplified medicine, since many other factors have also greatly influenced changes in the population's level of living in the rural areas. To measure success by health indices and statistics is also difficult, because not enough data are available from before the programme or since it began. A health survey and an in-depth study are needed to assess the degree of success through selected health indicators. An agreement was recently signed between the Ministry of Health and the International Development Research Centre, Canada, for an analysis of Venezuela's 10-year experience of simplified medicine. This evaluation, which will be carried out by the School of Public Health, University of Venezuela, is designed to provide answers to three main questions : the effectiveness of the services rendered ; the reactions of the communities served ; and the cost of the programme.

The health programme in Ivanjica, Yugoslavia [a]

Twenty years ago Ivanjica, an underdeveloped district in the Socialist Republic of Serbia, was connected with other parts of Serbia only by a macadam road via Afilje and Požega. In 1953 there were 13 kilometres of roads in good repair. Although the district is not waterless, no settlement except the small town of Ivanjica was supplied with pure drinking-water, and only Ivanjica and the surrounding villages had electricity. The only eight-year primary school was in Ivanjica, while the rest of the district had four-year schools.

The terrain is mountainous and intersected by deep streams and river beds. Of a total of 109 000 hectares, 16 250 are cultivated and 52 203 covered with forest. In the community there are 40 000 inhabitants, mostly farmers, living in 8000 households divided into 48 straggling settlements.

All health services were provided through a 62-bed hospital and an outpatient clinic in Ivanjica and two smaller outpatient clinics elsewhere in the district. Owing to the low standard of living and the low level of health and general culture, communicable and parasitic diseases were

---

[a] Case study prepared by Dr A. Nikolić, Dr L. Nikolić, and Dr B. Tomić.

common, and the inadequate diet of the inhabitants resulted in a great deal of illness.

In 1954 a new health centre, the House of Health, was established in Ivanjica. The most important tasks facing the newly organized health services were the initiation of thorough sanitation measures and the improvement of health education, the aim of which was the eradication and prevention of the many diseases that were prevalent in the area.

The health workers employed in the community were aware that the numerous problems of health protection could not be solved separately from the community's other problems. Multisectoral activities, with the object of improving living conditions, were carried out by physicians who worked predominantly on the spot, in direct contact with the village households. Thus the physicians were able to familiarize themselves with the conditions of the area and the various duties of health workers in a backward environment. The health workers had to be extremely persevering in their efforts to end superstition and other habits harmful to health that were woven into the lives of both rural and urban inhabitants.

The House of Health comprises the following services : a hygiene and epidemiological service ; a maternal and child health clinic ; a tuberculosis clinic ; a general practitioners' outpatient clinic with health stations in the district ; dental services ; and a laboratory and X-ray department.

In addition to the experience they gained working in the clinics and health stations, the first task of the health workers was to visit as many households as possible in order to study the living and working conditions, diet, health status, and the prevalence of disease. This study of hygienic conditions and health status proved very useful and later prompted a more elaborate study. In cooperation with the Serbian Institute of Health Education, an extensive field survey of health and hygienic conditions was carried out in 1963 on a sample of 5% of households. This provided valuable evidence of the adverse effect on the people's health status of the lack of education, various harmful habits and beliefs, and the low standard of living.

As a result, health education work is now accepted as an integral part of the health protection of the population. Originally it consisted of giving information and advice on health and disease. Lectures on health and disease were given at the adult education centre, in schools, as part of organized courses, and during health drives. Audiovisual aids were freely used. During outbreaks of epidemic diseases such as measles and whooping cough, information leaflets on protection and the care of sick children were distributed by the House of Health.

Encouraged by the success of health education, the health services made further efforts in health protection. Smaller health programmes were launched, involving the community in the improvement of their health standards. Instruction was by way of example rather than advice. The community was encouraged to construct hygienic houses, toilets, garbage disposal plants, farm buildings, and so on. In addition to being supplied with plans, each household was offered 600 kg of free cement.

The highest priority was given to the improvement of the water supply and of hygienic conditions in the village schools. Professional staff from the House of Health assisted local farmers and provided funds for the construction of waterworks and for spring-tapping, public fountains, washing facilities, and so forth. Priority was given to areas subject to epidemics of typhoid fever and other enteric infections and to areas distant from natural springs. Apart from the benefit to public health, the project created a greater feeling of social responsibility among the rural communities.

Special attention was paid to the improvement of school buildings. A total of 35 out of 37 buildings were improved with assistance from UNICEF, the Red Cross, and education workers. Dining halls and toilet facilities have been constructed with the help of the pupils' parents. Pupils were encouraged, with the help of parents and agronomists, to grow fruit and vegetables.

A small hydroelectric generating plant was constructed by the House of Health in the village of Kovilje to persuade the inhabitants of the advantages of electricity. It was later replaced by a larger plant supplying more households and a local school.

Outpatient clinics have become the focal point of villages. Newly constructed roads have made transport much easier. Full-time nurses are employed at the health stations, and physicians attend one or two days a week. In many centres their visits are timed to coincide with village market days, and villagers are shown films on health protection as well as on agriculture and other subjects.

The whole programme was coordinated by the House of Health through the community authorities, and financed by a local voluntary tax fund and special funds provided by the inhabitants. A hospital building in Ivanjica and many outpatient clinics in the district were constructed by volunteers.

The House of Health continues to run programmes in maternal and child health, tuberculosis control, health education, and environmental health. Its cooperation with local authorities and communities has resulted in the eradication of some communicable diseases, a reduction in the incidence of tuberculosis, the disappearance of criminal abortion, and a decline in the infant mortality rate.

The health insurance contributions of workers and farmers in Ivanjica have not always completely covered all the activities described, but many have cost very little.

Without any significant investment from the Republic or other communities, much was done in the 20 years from 1953 to 1973. Three hundred kilometres of rural roads were constructed and bus communications were established with even the remotest villages. Electricity was supplied to a large number of settlements and many new school buildings were erected. The intensive new construction has resulted in the improvement of housing conditions.

All these improvements have led to better health for the inhabitants of the district, to generally greater prosperity, and to faster development of the area.

Comprehensive rural health project, Jamkhed, India[a]

This project is designed to meet the basic health needs of a rural population of 40 000, mainly using local resources. It was initiated late in 1970 with its centre in Jamkhed village, Ahmednagar district, some 400 kilometres south-east of Bombay. Resources are scare in the area, which is agricultural; it has poor irrigation, and has suffered three consecutive years of drought.

The project works in close cooperation with the government health services system. The 30 villages it covers are well away from the primary health centre run by the government service. Four of the villages have government subcentres with auxiliary nurse-midwives. The project works with them, the project centre offering a referral centre for family planning and medical and surgical procedures beyond their scope.

The main objective is to meet basic health needs by providing the following services:

1. Maternal and child health services, including antenatal care, perinatal care, care at delivery, infant and child welfare, and family planning; immunization of children and mothers (smallpox, diphtheria, whooping cough, tetanus, poliomyelitis, BCG); prevention, detection, and correction of malnutrition; education and encouragement of the community to meet its own nutritional needs.

2. Health education in the community.

3. Diagnosis and treatment of simple common illnesses.

4. Medical and surgical emergencies.

5. Detection, prevention and control of such chronic illnesses as tuberculosis and leprosy.

6. Prevention and treatment of blindness.

7. Environmental health through the provision of safe drinking-water.

---

[a] Visit made and case study prepared by Dr R. H. O. Bannerman (WHO), Dr O. G. Beltram (WHO), Sister A. Cummins (UNICEF), and Dr V. Djukanovic (WHO).

In order to meet its objectives quickly and cheaply, the project has adopted the following strategy :

1. Extensive community participation.

2. Development of a training programme and utilization of village health workers.

3. Development of agriculture for the nutrition programme.

4. Provision of safe drinking-water by the sinking of deep tube wells with hand pumps in the most needy villages.

5. Organization of clinics at times determined by the activities of the community, not necessarily at the usual hours.

6. Health education—an important component of the project. Health education is given with the help of audiovisual aids such as flannelgraphs, flash cards, puppet shows and film strips. The community has helped by selecting people with histrionic talent for the purpose. A mobile educational exhibit is taken from village to village and mass health education is given with the help of puppet shows. This is followed up by village health workers talking to smaller groups. The aim is to create an awareness of the various health problems and their solutions.

General development scheme

In order to improve the quality of life, certain development programmes have been initiated by the local health authorities.

The agricultural projects include sheep-breeding (some 300 selected rams have been introduced to improve the flock) and an artificial insemination centre for cows. Twenty persons were each given 1000 rupees to start poultry farms. An oil mill and a seed improvement scheme were started but discontinued because of the severe drought.

The Government has also made housing loans available at 8% interest, repayable over 20 years. Many people have been unable to take up the loans because they have lacked the necessary initial capital.

The development priorities were defined as follows :

(a) development for agricultural production—water supply ;

(b) extension of electricity network fro irrigation pumps ;

(c) improved communication between villages—roads ;

(d) buildings :
— primary health centres, family planning centres
— storehouses for food grains
— schools
— other buildings.

Project administration

The project has a governing body composed of a chairman, secretary, treasurer and four other members. The two project senior physicians are ex-officio members. The nursing profession is represented, as is the WHO Regional Office for South-East Asia. The governing body approves the general policy and budget, and appoints the project director. The project director acts as chief executive and administrator and is assisted by an advisory committee composed of local leaders and representatives of the various groups—political parties and castes—in the community. The committee meets once or twice a year but a smaller working group meets every two or three months. The block development officer (a government official) is an ex-officio member of the advisory committee.

Project structure

A three-tier system of responsibility has been developed. The first line of contact with the community is the village health worker, selected by the communities themselves. This ensures effective communication with the villagers ; as she lives in the village herself, she is aware of their problems. She helps to trace target groups within the project's priorities, provides health education and first aid for the people, and works with the health team in house-to-house surveys. In-service training is given to these village health workers and, in addition, they receive training for two days a week at the project centre in Jamkhed. They receive an honorarium of one rupee per day.

The second tier consists of the nurse supervisor, medical social workers, auxiliary nurse-midwife, and leprosy and laboratory technicians, who work together in two teams and are responsible for supervising the village health workers. They visit each village once a week, carrying out house visits to detect malnutrition and communicable diseases (leprosy and tuberculosis), to look at expectant and lactating mothers, and to consider which couples are eligible for family planning. Appropriate promotional health talks (using audiovisual aids, including films) and programmes of, for example, immunization are arranged periodically. The members of the team are given in-service training together as a team, and each member has a specific role in the delivery of health care. The teaching emphasizes the project priorities. Ayurvedic and homoeopathic medical practitioners function independently in the area, but most cooperate actively in the project and two Ayurvedic doctors have been integrated into the project health teams.

The third tier consists of the project's two doctors, whose main functions are administration, supervision, training and the day-to-day running of the main centre at Jamkhed, which is the only medical facility in the area, and of the 30 project subcentres.

Of particular importance to the project's success in providing comprehensive services is the decision of the two staff physicians to allocate 30%

of their time for curative services, 30% for public health services, 20% for supervision, 10% for training, and 10% for self-education.

Finances

The project's total budget in 1973 was 520 000 rupees, of which 70% was derived from local fees and a government grant for family planning activities, and the other 30% from donations. It is hoped that by 1975 the project will be completely self-supporting. Curative services absorb 30% of the budget, while 60% goes on preventive services and promotional programmes. Administration and training activities account for the balance of 10%.

Project orientation and implementation

At the start of the project the main health problems were the rapid rate of population growth and high infant and child mortality rates. Chronic diseases such as tuberculosis and leprosy were common, as was malnutrition. Facilities for health care were poor and water was in short supply, so that agricultural activities were at a low ebb.

The project was initiated with the minimum of resources. There was close collaboration with the *dais* (traditional birth attendants), indigenous practitioners and the people working on government development programmes.

The initial aim was to reduce the birth rate from 40 to 30 per 1000 in six years and at the same time to halve the mortality rate of children aged under five years. Cases of tuberculosis and leprosy were to be identified and treated, primary health care was to be provided for the community, and training was to be organized for auxiliary staff.

In order to achieve basic health care coverage at low cost, the project design included the following innovations:

1. Agricultural support of the nutrition programme;

2. Deepening of wells for irrigation and the provision of safe drinking-water;

3. Use of fees derived from curative services to support promotive and preventive health programmes;

4. Training and use of village health workers;

5. Community participation and involvement in decision-making and support in the delivery of comprehensive health care;

6. Incorporation into the project of indigenous practitioners, Ayurvedic practitioners and *dais*.

House-to-house surveys were carried out to obtain baseline demographic, morbidity and mortality data, so that progress can be evaluated in relation to the stated objectives. Each of the 30 villages is visited at least once a month by a mobile health team.

Agricultural support of the nutrition programme

The project has identified itself fully with the population's felt needs. In order to implement its nutrition programme, the project lends tractors and other machinery to local farmers to plough and cultivate land that would otherwise lie fallow; in return, it receives 50% of the produce for the nutrition programme. The programme is also supported by small poultry and dairy farms, which provide eggs and milk.

Supplementary feeding programmes have been organized in 20 villages and are in full operation. In 1973, 1200 children received a regular daily morning meal.

Nutrition was a major problem during the drought, and children, expectant and nursing mothers, and tuberculosis patients were all given supplementary food.

The nutrition programme is fully self-supporting and receives no assistance from outside sources.

Deepening of wells for irrigation and provision of safe drinking-water

The drought badly affected agricultural production. To protect the community's 380 acres of land, 15 wells were deepened in 1973 to enable them to be used for irrigation purposes.

Lack of safe drinking-water in the area plays a large part in various illnesses. In 1973, tube wells were constructed in 21 villages, with the active participation of each village community.

Use of village health workers

The project seeks to find the methods of health care delivery best suited to the needs and resources of the area.

The village health worker—the first level in the Jamkhed system—is a member of the community and constantly in close contact with her fellow villagers; she therefore acts as the liaison officer between the community and the more educated nurse and other health workers. Delegation of each task to the least trained member of the team capable of performing the task satisfactorily is one way of overcoming the problem of inadequate manpower and financial resources.

The cultural gap between the city-educated health worker and the illiterate rural folk was soon noticed. Very often a patient, after listening to a physician or nurse, would more readily accept the advice of the illiterate watchman or sweeper of the health centre. This is because he identifies with another illiterate person and feels closer to him than to the educated and sophisticated physician or nurse. In one instance, a city-educated nurse who spent several months in a village could not persuade a single woman to undergo tubectomy, while an illiterate *dai* from the same village was able to refer 75 women for tubectomy within the same period. With these attitudes in mind, it was felt that the best way to get into the community and teach it to accept new methods and change its attitudes was to enlist the help of women from within the community.

The result has been, to take another instance, that in a relatively short period a village health worker has been able to persuade 200 women to accept antenatal care and has referred over 100 women for tubectomy. She is also able to follow up patients with tuberculosis and leprosy and persuade them to take treatment regularly from the clinic.

The village communities are asked to find women from amongst themselves who would be interested in joining the health care team. Usually, women with no household responsibilities volunteer for such work. They come to the health centre at Jamkhed on Saturdays and Sundays, and there are given regular classes on various health topics by the physicians, nurses and other workers in the health team. The women are mostly illiterate, and the bulk of the teaching is done with the help of flash cards and charts. The five priorities of the project are stressed and the village-level worker's role explained. Each class starts with a summary of the previous week's teaching and a discussion on the application of the knowledge gained to the work in the village. The women are also taught the use of flash cards so that they can use them in their promotional work. At the end of 1973, 8 workers were being trained by this method and the results appeared very encouraging.

Community participation

From the start, community participation has been an essential part of the project. The community in Jamkhed is poor and lacks good housing, electricity, and running water. However, it provided simple accommodation for the project and staff and donated land and buildings for the work, not only in the main centre but also in the villages. In all the villages the community assists voluntarily in the preparation of food for the nutrition programme. In addition, it contributes to the buildings of roads to give health team workers better access to the villages. A youth organization collects blood for the health centre and villages and is particularly active in mass mobilization for immunization and in other public health activities. The community is involved not only in carrying out the programme but also in making the decisions. It feels strongly that the health centre and the whole health services system are a part of its own system and considers all the project's problems as its own. In effect, it has developed a strong sense of belonging and involvement.

The incorporation of indigenous practitioners in the project, with the facilities for referral offered to them, is clearly an advantage to the community. Ayurvedic practitioners are members of the staff and the local Ayurvedic practitioners cooperate closely.

Achievements

The Jamkhed project has had considerable success in realizing its objectives in a relatively short time, despite the fact that the project area suffered a drought during the two years up to 1973. Indeed, this was an additional challenge that the project faced successfully. The achievements have been considerable in a number of specific fields :

1. Mass immunization (diphtheria, pertussis, tetanus, BCG and poliomyelitis). Mass vaccination programmes are regularly carried out for children aged under five years. BCG is given up to the age of 20 years, since tuberculosis is one of the major problems.

2. Leprosy and tuberculosis detection and treatment. These are being continuously developed. The number of second visits is rising constantly, possibly as a result of effective health education among patients. The number of new patients with leprosy and tuberculosis decreased slightly in 1973, probably because of detection activities earlier in the year rather than lower morbidity.

3. Rapid progress has been made in maternal and child health and family planning. The number of second visits to the antenatal clinic increased from month to month throughout 1973, doubling by the middle of the year and continuing to increase. Full information about the number of women who have made these repeat visits in the past, if it were available, would permit further conclusions regarding the efficiency of antenatal care. The number of first clinic attendances showed monthly variations in 1973, with a slight but obvious increase over the year.

4. As to the prevention of pregnancy, the number of newcomers receiving oral contraceptives each month fluctuated from 10 to 20 at first, increasing to 50–60 in June and July 1973. The number of old acceptors increased from 290 in January to 480 in December. Although great progress was made between 1971 and the end of 1973, the service has still not sufficiently covered the female population or reached all groups equally. Among women acceptors in 1973 there was a higher percentage of women with two and three children, possibly because the idea of an optimal family size is spreading via health education, or the women were more receptive to health advice at that stage in life. Information on the total female population

76

according to parity will be needed for further analysis of existing problems and development of the family planning services. Tubectomy was performed mostly on women with two, three and four children. There has been no appreciable change in the last two years ; the number of women requesting tubectomy has not increased greatly nor has the parity of the women in 1973 changed essentially from 1971.

5. One thousand two hundred children had supplementary feeding in 1973 and there have been enormous improvements in water supply and irrigation ; 15 irrigation wells and 18 safe drinking-water supplies have been constructed. The figures for curative services during the first half of 1973 were : outpatients 4040 ; second visits 5580 ; inpatients 627.

Conclusions

Within the terms of reference of the present study, it seems clear that the project has achieved remarkable success. In a very short period of time the target population has been fully provided with primary health care services, and these services have been effectively integrated with services to meet the agricultural and water supply needs of the people. All the services are extensively and enthusiastically used and financially sustained by the community.

Several factors seem relevant to this success. One of the most important is that the project is based on the recognition, particularly by the project leaders, of the priorities determined by the community. To the community, health is not a number one priority ; agriculture, water supplies and housing are more important. The project has therefore identified itself firmly with agricultural improvement, acquiring a tractor to be hired out to farmers and providing assistance in dairy and poultry farming and irrigation schemes. In effect, it appears that in such communities, which have a low economic status and per capita income, doctors and health services will need to identify themselves with the community's priorities in order to fulfil health objectives.

The effective use of the health team approach, with responsibility delegated to the least trained of the team capable of performing any particular task, makes full coverage a reality. The awakening within the community of concern for its own health needs also contributes greatly to success.

Finally, the enormous dedication of the health team and the dynamic leadership of the two doctors through whose efforts and initiative the project was begun have contributed greatly to the overall success of the project.

Use of village health workers and trained traditional birth attendants in the Department of Maradi, Niger [a]

Background

The Department of Maradi lies in the dry savannah in the south of the Republic of Niger. It has about 700 000 inhabitants, of whom about 11% are nomads (Fulanis and Tuaregs) and 88% are settled Hausas, in an area of about 38 500 km². Annual population growth is estimated at 2.7%. Administratively, the Department is divided into six *arrondissements* or districts and one municipality (Maradi). Its road network is poor. The local economy is mainly agricultural.

The crude mortality rate is estimated at 27 per 1000, while the infant mortality rate is between 250 and 300 per 1000 births. Malnutrition is common at the weaning age, and hygienic conditions are unsatisfactory. The main causes of sickness are infectious and parasitic diseases, particularly malaria, gastrointestinal disorders, and eye and skin infections.

The health services in Maradi Department include : the headquarters of the departmental health services ; a departmental hospital ; a mobile team for the Department consisting of two squads for vaccination and the detection of disease ; the Maradi urban health area ; and six health districts. The urban area and districts have financial autonomy, health activities being financed from the local and not the national budget.

In the health districts there are 17 rural dispensaries, three medical (health) centres with a total of 82 beds, and three maternity hospitals (32 beds). The bed/population ratio is 1 : 6000 when the health services of Maridi municipality are excluded. In the next five-year development plan (1975–1979), one additional rural dispensary, three medical centres (60 beds) and three maternity hospitals (24 beds) are planned. The privately funded health infrastructure is limited to one leprosarium and one rural dispensary.

The personnel working in the local public health services in 1974 consist of eight medical officers (four working in the hospital in Maradi, three living in the town but working in the Department, and one in Tessaoua), one dentist (in the hospital in Maradi), three midwives (two working in the hospital and one in the Department), 24 registered nurses (six in the hospital, the rest working in the Department), 57 certified nurses and 16 auxiliary nurses. In the rural areas, as a result of the uneven distribution of health personnel, there is only one medical officer for every 170 000 inhabitants and one nurse or auxiliary nurse for 9430 inhabitants. The catchment areas of rural dispensaries are confined to a 10–15 kilometre radius.

---

[a] Visit made and case study prepared by Dr E. Kalimo (WHO), Mr J. F. Barres (UNICEF), and Dr M. Torfs (WHO).

Less than 15% of patients in the Department are covered by the health services, which means that 85% of them take care of their own health problems with the help of either native doctors or traditional healers. Apart from insufficient manpower and facilities, this lack of coverage is also the outcome of the passive attitude of the health personnel. For example, most dispensary nurses expect patients to make their way to the dispensary. The concepts of preventive medicine remain in the realm of theory, while maternal and child health and health education are seldom part of nurses' everyday activities. Their inertia and lack of interest can apparently be attributed to their ignorance of local public health problems, as their training is almost exclusively geared to curative medicine.

Extension of health protection of the rural population

Although the coverage of the population is still poor, several activities have been undertaken since 1966, on the joint initiative of the departmental health services and the rural development services,[a] that have considerably improved the local situation. The strategy chosen and gradually put into effect had three main elements :

1. Initiation of better health coverage through joint information efforts by the rural development services, the education and literacy services and the health services, supported by the political party ;

2. Health protection through the setting up of village health teams consisting of two voluntary part-time village health workers and some traditional birth attendants, who become the frontline link between villagers and the health services ;

3. Orientation of the auxiliary health worker towards rural health through the practice of comprehensive health care and dynamic participation in educational, supervisory and technical activities.

This strategy, implemented exclusively by national personnel, is the result of research during field operations and dialogue with the local population. It is based on :

— in-depth study and knowledge of the sociocultural and economic conditions of the areas to be covered ;

— the organization of multisectoral groups to discuss local health problems and ways of tackling them at the lowest cost ; in these groups, high-level representatives of health, rural development,

---

[a] The rural development services (*animation rurale*) form an administrative, technical and educational structure, usually part of the Ministry of Development (Rural Branch) but sometimes of the Ministry of Education, whose function is to motivate people to participate in rural development activities.

literacy and education services and the ruling political party participate in discussions chaired by the highest administrative authority
(the *sous-préfet* or *préfet*) ;

— continuous communication with and information and sensitization
of the rural population with a view to gradually increasing its
motivation and direct involvement.

The contacts with the population through the rural development and
health services aim at :

(*a*) explanation of the objectives of the community participation now
proposed and the role the villagers have to play in it ;

(*b*) selection of village health workers by the villagers themselves ;

(*c*) installation of the village health workers (with elementary pharmacy)
and/or traditional birth attendants after completion of their training ;

(*d*) annual retraining of the village health workers in order to maintain
and improve their skills.

Village health workers and the village pharmacies

The choice of village health workers is left entirely to the villagers
themselves, provided that certain basic criteria are fulfilled, for example,
that they should be volunteers, live in the village, and be prepared to undergo
the necessary training.

The villagers chosen by the community are given 10 days of essentially
practice-based training, which is organized at the nearest dispensary or
health centre by the nurse in charge, assisted by the chief nurse in charge
of the health district. The courses cover : general health concepts, emergencies and referrals, epidemic diseases, health education (including nutrition),
elementary health care, environmental sanitation, and some record-keeping.

The main aim is to prevent diseases and wounds from becoming complicated while awaiting referral of the patient and to refer patients who
cannot be treated with the elementary means available to better equipped
health facilities in time. Village health workers are also intended to improve
environmental conditions in the village.

Health information is constantly exchanged with the population and
village health workers through close and regular supervision by the auxiliary
nurse in charge of the nearest dispensary or health centre. In turn, this nurse
receives support from the higher echelons.

Each year the village health workers already in service attend a 10-day
refresher course which will gradually include new items related to local
health needs, e.g., the treatment of malnutrition and the preparation of
weaning foods. The cost of these courses is about Fr. CFA 1500 (US $6)
per person.

Experience has shown that trained village health workers are capable of treating patients suffering from most locally common diseases such as malaria and diarrhoea, superficial wounds, and some skin and eye diseases. For this purpose they receive small quantities of basic drugs : an antiseptic, eye drops, and chloroquine, aspirin and guanidine tablets. Some of these drugs are sold to the patients at fixed low prices, the money collected being used to restock the pharmacy. Other drugs, including mercurochrome, argyrol and methylene blue, are distributed free of charge.

The first allocation of drugs to each village pharmacy is paid for out of the health district budget. Replacements for the drugs are paid for by the villagers, while the dispensary nurse supervising health activities at the village level is responsible for arranging supplies. Village drug sales average Fr. CFA 500 (US $2) per month.

Each village has a health management team, which controls the administrative functioning of the village health workers and their pharmacy. The training of the members of this team takes three days. The chairman of the team assists in all financial matters, while the treasurer keeps the stocks of the pharmacy, purchases new drugs, and records all financial transactions. Since the village health worker—the third element in the team—is a volunteer, his only reward for the health work he performs is that the villagers provide his day-to-day subsistence (mainly food). In addition, he probably receives some gifts from the villagers in accordance with tradition.

Achievements and prospects

At the end of 1973, 109 villages in Maradi Department were served by 218 village health workers. By mid-1974, the number of village pharmacies had increased by 20 to 129. During 1973, 136 129 consultations were given by the village health workers in 88 villages (no reports were available for 21 villages), representing 12.8% of all consultations given in Maradi Department by health organization workers.

The resources available from local health services will allow the scheme to be extended in a reasonable and planned fashion to 30 more villages each year ; this will entail training 60 new village health workers and setting up 30 village pharmacies.

An interesting aspect of this programme has been its impact on the training, mobilization and motivation of other health personnel, and particularly the auxiliary dispensary nurse. As he is responsible for supervising village health workers, he has been compelled to improve his knowledge and to become more involved ; he is now a trainer instead of the simple dispenser of drugs that he was previously.

The rate of extension of the scheme is slow in view of the limited financial resources and of the scarcity of auxiliary personnel working at the supervisory level. Ideally two auxiliary nurses should staff each dispensary in order to pay supervisory visits to all village health workers regularly—once or even twice a month—and meanwhile to keep the dispensary operating for patients living in its neighbourhood. Because the scheme is being extended so slowly, drastic changes are needed in the strategy for the development of health services as a whole. Among the problems still to be solved are manpower training and the distribution of financial resources so that they do not go only to existing health establishments.

Training of traditional birth attendants

Traditionally, the role of the traditional birth attendant was limited to burying the placenta and giving the most elementary care to the child and mother. Surveys in Maradi Department have shown that despite the presence of traditional birth attendants, the mortality rate among women and children is high both during and after delivery as a result of either pregnancy complications or neglected infections.

It was decided that the performance of traditional birth attendants should be improved by some training, to enable them to be more active and effective even before the delivery, to apply higher standards of hygiene, to refer complicated cases to health centres or maternity hospitals, and to register the newborn. Traditional birth attendants are selected for training in a similar way to village health workers. They are trained for 15 days in the maternity ward of a health centre or in the district rural hospital.

The training is essentially practical and relates to all phases of childbirth, including prenatal and postnatal care. Its objectives are : to reduce infant mortality ; to improve standards of hygiene during delivery ; to educate the mother in better nutrition during pregnancy and weaning ; to obtain a statistical record of births ; and thus to compensate for the scarcity of maternity hospitals.

At the end of the course the knowledge acquired is tested and only the most capable traditional birth attendants are appointed. They then receive a basic UNICEF midwifery kit with some drugs and equipment. They are supervised during visits at monthly intervals by the nurse in charge of the nearest dispensary, who supplies them with drugs. The cost of training each traditional birth attendant is about Fr. CFA 4620 (US $21), equipment and supplies included. UNICEF has so far borne the cost of most of this training.

Although the traditional birth attendant is in principle a voluntary worker, it is customary for her to receive a gift after each delivery. The size of the gift depends on local circumstances and traditions.

Achievements and prospects

In 1973, 1071 deliveries were assisted by the 241 trained traditional birth attendants working in Maradi Department ; this represented 28% of all deliveries recorded in maternity homes in the Department. There were

65 referrals. There has been a dramatic improvement in the hygienic conditions in which deliveries take place. In addition, some of the birth attendants already play a more active role in the prenatal and postnatal consultations organized in a number of dispensaries or maternity units, and traditional practices during weaning are gradually being changed.

In 1974, it was planned to train 91 traditional birth attendants covering 32 villages. The intention was to train a selection of younger but nevertheless acceptable women who would presumably have a higher capacity for assimilation, and to widen the scope of the activities of the trained traditional birth attendants.

The pace of extension of this training scheme also depends on the supervisory capacity of the dispensaries and health centres. Additional assistance might be obtained if the means at the disposal of the departmental mobile teams could be increased or district mobile teams could be established.

Health and nutrition education

Through the joint efforts of the rural development, health and education services, a departmental workshop has been set up to provide elementary support to village health workers and trained traditional birth attendants (e.g., flannelgraphs, booklets) for activities in health and nutrition education directly related to their respective functions. Teachers and other professional personnel also receive this equipment and take part in the same activities. Nutritional health education covers mainly weaning problems, for which cheap and locally available solutions are needed.

Replicability of the schemes

The achievements of the schemes to establish village health workers with their village pharmacies and train traditional birth attendants in Maradi Department are the result of intersectoral teamwork leading to the motivation and active participation of the villagers in activities for health protection. The extension of the schemes to other departments of Niger is proposed and a national evaluation of their progress is under consideration.

The replicability of the Maradi approach will depend mainly on whether a number of avoidable or at least reducible constraints can be overcome, among which the motivation of decision-makers at intermediate and central level is not the least. Manpower needs are still increasing and the development of the system is handicapped by lack of finance. Transport, equipment, supplies and drugs are badly needed, and UNICEF is actively helping here. Experience has shown that the schemes can lead to a better coverage of the rural population provided that they are programmed realistically and rationally in the light of conditions in each village. The continuing involvement of multisectoral service teams specially designed to assist the communities in the development process is also required.

Indigenous systems of medicine : Ayurvedic medicine in India [a]

The belief that illness arises from supernatural causes and indicates the displeasure of ancestral gods and evil spirits or is the effect of black magic is still held by many communities in developing countries. To deal with such causes, indigenous healers undertake elaborate exorcising rituals on behalf of the sick and mentally afflicted. In some countries, indeed, diseases have been classified into three broad categories—those curable by indigenous medicine, those curable by modern medicine, and those that are self-limiting and not affected by either indigenous or modern medicine.

Some kind of health care therefore exists everywhere, but though it may be psychologically acceptable to the individual it may be largely ineffective or even harmful as far as the illness is concerned. This is not to deny that the classical clinical approach to modern scientific medicine, particularly in the developing countries, is not infrequently biased, incomplete and, indeed, potentially harmful because it pays no heed to sociocultural factors. In this respect, the great traditions of Arabic, Chinese, and Hindu medicine require consideration, because they are relevant to the urgent problem of improving health care, in particular the problem of providing total health care coverage for the population.

Ayurvedic medicine may be taken as an example of the efficacy of a fairly well organized indigenous system of medicine and health care. It originated in India and has been practised there and in neighbouring countries for some 3000 years ; and it continues to be supported and used by most of the people living in those countries. As an integral part of Indian culture it cannot be ignored.

It is estimated that about 80% of the population living in the rural areas of India and neighbouring countries have confidence in and use the Ayurvedic system. Nevertheless, most of the governments support modern medical science and are uncertain how to use Ayurvedic practitioners. Some of them, however, are studying the question of how indigenous systems could best be utilized for more effective or total health coverage.

Some provincial and state governments in India have interested themselves in the use of Indian medicine in the rural areas. Schools and colleges of Indian medicine were opened in various states to train competent practitioners of Indian medicine and give them a good working knowledge of western medicine, so that they could provide the rural population with a comprehensive medical service. It was also proposed to promote research and eventually to integrate Indian and modern medicine, with a health team consisting of doctors, physical training experts, sanitarians, physiotherapists, nurses, and midwives.

---

[a] Visit made and case study prepared by Dr R. H. O. Bannerman (WHO), Sister A. Cummins (UNICEF), Dr V. Djukanovic (WHO), and Dr U Ko Ko (WHO).

A Central Council of Indian Medicine was established by the Government of India in 1971. Among its main functions are the recognition of qualifications in Indian medicine, the prescription of minimum standards of education in Indian medicine, and the maintenance of a central register of practitioners. The Council has established minimum standards and a curriculum for undergraduate and postgraduate education.

Categories of Ayurvedic practitioners

Ayurvedic practitioners in India can be broadly divided into four categories. The first, of whom there are about 7000, are those who have received a fully integrated training in modern and Ayurvedic systems of medicine and can use both in their practice. The second, about 43 000 in all, are those who are trained mostly in Ayurvedic medicine in Ayurvedic institutions but also have some elementary knowledge of modern medicine. They practise mostly in smaller rural communities, using Ayurvedic medicine in general and modern drugs mainly in emergencies. The third, about 150 000 in all, are Ayurvedic practitioners without formal training who have obtained diplomas in Ayurveda after correspondence courses and examinations. They practise only Ayurvedic medicine. Into the fourth category fall those without either institutional training or qualifications who practise Ayurvedic medicine after experience as apprentices with Ayurvedic physicians. There are about 200 000 in this category and they practise in the rural areas ; they include the traditional birth attendants called *dais*.

Proposed integration into the national health services

How can these 400 000 fully trained, half-trained, and untrained Ayurvedic physicians and other indigenous health workers be best used to provide health care for the people ? At present the rural areas in India do not have adequate health care. The ratio of doctors to the population in urban areas is 1 : 1200, but in rural areas it is 1 : 11 000 and in some remote areas even more unfavourable. To incorporate Ayurvedic physicians and indigenous health workers into the government health services might completely revolutionize medical and health care in India, which has a rural population of about 500 million people.

It is worth emphasizing that nearly 90% out of the total of 400 000 Ayurvedic practitioners of different types serve the rural areas. The remaining 10% work in the cities and towns, where most of them have lucrative practices. The rural population in general is said to prefer physicians fully trained in both modern and Ayurvedic medicine.

Practice of Ayurvedic medicine

Ayurveda practises an integrated psychosomatic approach to health. Like modern medicine, it has two major components—preventive and curative.

1. *Prevention in Ayurveda*

Personal and social hygiene. In Ayurveda early rising and the regular daily performance of certain prescribed routines are recommended. Evacuation of the bowels and cleaning of the teeth are followed by Yoga exercises, then by a bath, prayers, a meal according to a regulated diet, work, adequate rest, and sleep. These prescribed daily routines are adjusted to the country, the climatic conditions, and the environment in which the person is living. Ayurveda also lays down that his social behaviour should be such as not to interfere with the physical or mental health of others.

Rejuvenating measures. Two methods are described in Ayurveda : *rasayana*, or rejuvenation, and *vajukarana*, or the use of aphrodisiacs. The main aims of *rasayana* therapy are : the prevention of aging and an increase in longevity ; improvement of the memory and intelligence ; the promotion of immunity and bodily resistance to disease and decay ; the imparting of lustre and vitality to the body ; and the maintenance of the optimum strength of the body and sense organs. To achieve these desired effects, many well-known herbs are given either singly or in combination for prolonged periods, and certain exercises and other measures are prescribed. The various Yoga practices are commonly used for the purpose.

Practice of Yoga. The word " Yoga " means " union ", and its exponents claim that by the continuous practice of Yoga a perfect union of body, mind, and soul can be attained, leading to complete tranquillity and peace. Yoga practices should be selected to suit the individual, who should, for example, carry out a few postural exercises, a few breathing exercises, and then some type of meditation. The practice does not take more than 30 minutes and therefore can be done either in the morning or in the evening.

A recent study of volunteers undertaking various postural and breathing exercises for six months found a significant increase in their vital capacity and a decrease in their heart and respiration rate, as well as significant decreases in their body weight, blood sugar, and blood cholesterol. Their urinary excretion of corticoids and testosterone was increased. Their memory was improved and they were less neurotic. Those who practised meditation showed a significant decrease in plasma cortisol, urinary corticoids, and urinary nitrogen excretion, and a significant increase in the blood levels of the different neurohumours and related enzymes. The findings indicated that after meditation the subjects were physically stable and resilient and mentally very active. The practice of Yoga may prove an effective method of keeping physically and mentally fit.

It has also been observed that the regular practice of Yoga helps patients to overcome the early stages of asthma, diabetes mellitus, thyrotoxicosis, and hypertension.

2. Curative treatment in Ayurveda

Internal medicine and therapeutics. Drugs play an important part in treatment. They are used mainly to eliminate causative factors by inducing vomiting or purging, and they include various types of enema and inhalation. Elimination is carried out as far as possible before drug therapy, rejuvenation therapy, or surgical treatment is instituted.

An example of treatment according to Ayurvedic principles is that for rheumatoid arthritis. The theory is that in this disease all the bodily humours become vitiated and settle in the joints. First various eliminating procedures are carried out, then specific drug therapy is instituted, e.g. with the gum *guggulu* (from the tree *Boswellia serrata*) and its preparations.

The second type of treatment aims at neutralizing morbid humours by giving appropriate drugs, diet, and physiotherapy. A large number of herbal, mineral, and biological preparations are used singly or in combination, depending upon their pharmacodynamic properties. In the management of hemiplegia following a cerebrovascular accident, for example, Ayurvedic physicians give specific drugs to stimulate regeneration of the peripheral nerves ; purified nux vomica and other drugs with similar properties are administered for prolonged periods, mostly in the form of powders, liquid extracts, tinctures, decoctions, and tablets. Attempts have been made in recent years to standardize the preparation of these drugs and to isolate their active principles. The derivative of one of them, *Rauwolfia serpentina*, has been extensively used all over the world, and other useful drugs will doubtless come into widespread use in the near future.

In addition to drugs, Ayurveda attaches great importance to diet. A large variety of dietetic preparations are used for the maintenance of the nutritional status of patients during illness. In acute gastroenteritis in children the modern physician would advise parenteral restoration of the fluid balance, but Ayurvedic physicians try to maintain the fluid balance by planning the oral fluid intake and administering appropriate antiemetic and antidiarrhoeal treatment. They recommend specific fluids such as whey water, boiled rice water, and fresh coconut water, as well as specific fruit juices with astringent properties such as apple juice and pomegranate juice. They forbid milk in such cases.

Ayurveda has a prescribed treatment for all types of acute and chronic illness. The treatment appears to be effective in chronic metabolic diseases such as diabetes mellitus, atherosclerosis, and lipid storage diseases. Arthritis, gastrointestinal and urinary tract diseases, asthma, allergy, some skin diseases, some chronic diseases of the nervous system, and some mental ailments are also amenable to Ayurvedic treatment. Many patients with diseases that do not readily respond to modern treatment have benefited greatly from Ayurvedic treatment.

On the other hand, there is no effective Ayurvedic method for managing such acute emergencies as perforated peptic ulcer. Here the Ayurvedic physician needs to make a correct diagnosis and refer the patient to a specialist, and it is essential that he should be able to differentiate these acute emergencies and to take prompt action.

Medicines for external application. In addition to internal medicines, Ayurveda prescribes a large number of medicines for external use in the form of pastes, medicated oils for massage, medicated baths, gargles, and powders. The efficacy of medicated oils for treating some joint and neuro-muscular disorders is well known, as is the treatment of burns with specific preparations, Ointments prepared from papaya juice are applied to early superficial burns to produce a gradual débridement of devitalized and dead tissue. When débridement is complete and healthy granulation tissue appears, healing is promoted by the local application of medicated ghee prepared from the flower of the *jati*, the Spanish jasmine. In extensive burns such treatment is supplemented with skin grafting to replace lost tissue.

Surgical treatment. Ayurveda describes in detail various surgical condi-tions and their management, including different types of fracture, urinary stones, piles, fistulae, goitre, lymphadenitis, hernia, and hydrocele. Other treatment described includes plastic operations such as rhinoplasty and otoplasty and the ambulatory treatment of fistula in ano using corrosive threads in preference to the extensive excision of fistulous tracks, which requires confinement in bed for several days and involves the risk of second-ary infection.

Psychosomatic treatment. Although Ayurveda describes treatment for specific diseases, the Ayurvedic physician is required to adapt the composi-tion and dosage of the drugs employed, the diet, and rest to the psychoso-matic constitution of the individual patient and also to the relative pre-dominance of vitiated humours in the disease process. For mental disorders special prayers and offerings are made to the gods in order to allay the harmful effects of evil spirits on the patients and their families.

Training of Ayurvedic physicians

Nearly 100 Ayurvedic colleges exist in India and they have so far trained some 50 000 Ayurvedic physicians, Most of these qualified physicians have not only a good basic knowledge of Ayurvedic medicine but also an adequate knowledge of modern medicine. There can be no doubt that, if additional short-term refresher courses were provided for them, they would be eminently equipped to meet the primary medical and health care needs of rural populations. It is now becoming clear that the ultimate solution to the health problems of the developing nations is a fully integrated type of training embracing the essential principles of both indigenous systems of medicine and modern medical science, so that practitioners can serve the rural populations effectively and understandingly and at relatively low cost.

Postgraduate training. An integrated postgraduate medical education system has been developed at the Banaras Hindu University, Varanasi. The College of Ayurveda was established at the University as early as 1927 and instituted a five-year integrated training programme in Indian medicine and modern medicine and surgery leading to the award of the degree of A.M.S. and later of A.B.M.S. (Ayurveda Bachelor of Medicine and Surgery). A training programme in all fields of medical science was developed, but in 1960 the undergraduate course in Ayurveda was discontinued, the state and central governments having refused to recognize the A.B.M.S. as equivalent to an M.B., B.S. However, the importance of Indian medicine was fully appreciated and a postgraduate training course in Indian medicine started in 1963 at the College of Medical Sciences of the Banaras Hindu University.

Three years later the Postgraduate Institute of Indian Medicine was founded. A three-year postgraduate course leading to a doctorate in Ayurvedic medicine (D.Ay.M.) was established, admission to which is open to graduates in both Ayurvedic and modern medicine. In the first year after graduation in Ayurveda the doctor has to undergo training in applied aspects of modern medical subjects, while the graduate in modern medicine has to study the basic principles of Ayurveda. The next two years are devoted to studies and clinical and laboratory research in any one of the five Ayurvedic specialties. At the end of the two-year period the candidate submits a thesis and is examined in two papers on the subject of his specialization. There is an additional paper on classical Ayurvedic texts and another on an allied modern subject. This training programme enables students to acquire knowledge in both Indian and modern medicine and to undertake and analyse original research.

Since 1966 a course for a Ph.D. degree in Ayurveda has been developed, with a view to promoting advanced research in Ayurvedic subjects.

The Indian Medicine Unit of the Institute of Medical Sciences contains six departments dealing with :

(1) The principles of Ayurveda.

(2) Dravyaguna (properties of medicinal substances, materia medica, pharmacology).

(3) Kaya chikitsa (therapeutics, general medicine).

(4) Shalaya shalkya (surgery, major and minor).

(5) Prasuti tantra (obstetrics and gynaecology).

(6) Medicinal chemistry.

The university also runs a regular course in modern medicine for the training of students for the M.B., B.S., M.D., and M.S. degrees, the admission requirements being the same as for other medical colleges. Students undergo a five-year course including Ayurvedic medicine and surgery, and follow it up by a six-month internship. It is generally held that the M.B., B.S. course should include the essentials of Ayurvedic medicine so that practitioners should be better equipped for health work in India.

Research

In the field of applied research the Institute of Medical Sciences has made several contributions to knowledge about the therapeutic value of Ayurvedic drugs by determining the mode of action, isolating the active principles, and assessing the effective dosage and toxicity. An anabolic steroid isolated from *Cissus quadrangularis* has been studied extensively to determine its role in fracture healing. A catabolic steroid has been isolated that is said to be highly effective in the prevention and treatment of hyperlipidaemia and its complications, including atherosclerosis and coronary thrombosis. The herbal substances *jati ghrit* and *kshar sutra* have also been standardized for wound healing and for the treatment of fistula in ano by means of suitably impregnated sutures passed through the fistular tract. Other drugs that have been studied include *Picrorrhiza kurrooa* for the treatment of liver diseases, *Allium sativum* for the control of hypercholesterolaemia and heart diseases, *Semicarpus anacardium* for worm infestations and arthritis, *tambul* for heart diseases, and *punarnava* for urinary diseases.

There is also an urgent need for research on Yoga, which has generated worldwide interest in recent years.

To determine how best to provide the rural population with health care efficiently and cheaply, pilot research schemes will be needed in different parts of the country, using local resources including health manpower.

Examples of Ayurvedic practice

An example of a private Ayurvedic clinic is that in Narayanpur, some 50 kilometres from Varanasi. The clinic is operated by a couple of Ayurvedic physicians, both graduates of Banaras Hindu University. The senior partner specializes in ophthalmology, undertakes refractions, and dispenses lens and spectacle frames. The private nursing home has 10 beds with a small but well equipped operating theatre and the cases treated include entropion, pterygium, cataract, rectal fistula, haemorrhoids, hernia, and open fractures. The wife is responsible for minor obstetric and gynaecological procedures such as forceps delivery, dilatation and curettage, episiotomy, and repair. Another Ayurvedic practitioner in the same village also has an active outpatient clinic and specializes in dentistry.

The team leader of a government dispensary in a suburb of Varanasi is an Ayurvedic practitioner. Four beds are provided for the treatment and observation of patients. The dispensary is well organized and the small pharmacy store contains both Ayurvedic and modern therapeutic agents, including antibiotics. Infectious diseases are treated and notified to the public health authorities. Acute medical and surgical emergencies beyond the scope of the local facilities are referred to the central hospital for treatment and subsequently returned to the dispensary for follow-up and outpatient treatment.

In a survey of indigenous medical practitioners in the rural areas of five Indian states in 1973, all persons practising any system of curative medicine without recognized qualifications in modern medicine were interviewed. It was reported that only 7.4% of the practitioners had obtained institutional training and qualifications and that 65.6% were unqualified and could be classified as " quacks " or " unfit to practise ". The remainder had followed a correspondence course. Many were prescribing allopathic medicines and had no training in modern medicine. The tendency was for these practitioners to be located in the large villages ; the majority of the smaller villages with a population of 3000 or less had no resident practitioner. The coverage was between 5.5 and 9.8 indigenous practitioners per 10 000 of the rural populations surveyed.

Conclusions

Recognition of indigenous systems by the governments of the countries in which they exist would help in improving the quality of the practitioners and promoting knowledge of the systems. Surveys indicate that the practitioners urgently need additional training to improve their efficiency and usefulness. The training programmes should be structured to meet the special needs of the different categories of indigenous practitioner, and priority should be given in them to community and public health practice. Practitioners of modern medicine and undergraduate students also require instruction in indigenous systems as appropriate, in order to improve their knowledge of them and bring about the necessary changes in their attitude to them. Only in these ways can indigenous systems be integrated into government-sponsored health services. In India, an estimated 400 000 indigenous practitioners are functioning—mostly in the rural areas—and they could probably be developed and utilized to provide full coverage of the rural population. In the light of these considerations, the development of mass services or total health coverage for rural communities appears to be a more realistic aim than once seemed possible.

Nigeria : Use of two-way radio in the delivery of health services[a]

Improved communication through two-way radio can help to solve some health service problems in the rural areas of most developing countries. These problems include : lack of consultation and referral facilities ; poor supervision of the staff; lack of further professional training ; feelings of isolation and neglect among the staff in outlying posts ; inadequate supplies of drugs and other requirements ; rigid or restricted transport facilities ; and insufficient information about health service needs and the ability of dispensaries and other outlying posts to meet them.

The two-way radio system in North-Western State, Nigeria, is only one possible application of two-way radios ; similar schemes are in effect in other African countries as well as in other continents. Many of the two-way radio schemes are accompanied by a flying doctor service, since the former is obviously a prerequisite of the latter. The history of two-way radio systems goes back to the mid-1920s, when a scheme was started as a component of a flying doctor service in Australia.

The present study focused on the Nigerian scheme for two main reasons. First, the Government was interested in it from the beginning and later ran the scheme, whereas most of the other two-way radio schemes are financed from voluntary funds or foreign aid. Secondly, the Nigerian scheme was operated on scanty resources, a situation common in the health services of most developing countries.

The Federal Republic of Nigeria, which had a population of about 80 million in November 1973, is divided into 12 states. North-Western State is one of the largest states in Nigeria, and at the same time one of the poorest and least developed. Its area of 16 900 km² contained a population of approximately 7 232 000 at the end of 1972, of whom about half were under 15 years of age. Some 85% live in rural areas, the state being predominantly agricultural.

Basic medical care at the village level is provided in the state by dispensaries, of which there were 129 in 1973. Staffed by a trained (male) medical auxiliary and two untrained staff members, their function is mainly curative. They are administered and supervised by the local authorities, but the state Ministry of Health has a statutory right of technical supervision over them. Supplies are provided by the local authorities from the State Medical Store.

In 1973, there were about 50 000 people to each dispensary, including dispensaries run by the missions. It is estimated that an additional 360 dispensaries in the state by 1980 would not result in an even distribution

---

[a] Visit made and case study prepared by Dr A. Adeniyi-Jones (UNICEF), Dr E. Kalimo (WHO), and Dr M. Torfs (WHO).

in rural areas, so that special arrangements to reach sections of the population without health care would still be necessary.

As the area of the North-Western State is large, health institutions may be far from supervisors. Although most of the outlying dispensaries can be reached by a vehicle of the Land Rover type, travel, even by car, to the institutions to be supervised would take days. Dispensaries do not usually have access to a telephone.

The two-way radio scheme

A two-way radio communication scheme was established as a component of a flying doctor service in Northern Nigeria in 1963. The base station was at the Gusau Central Hospital, with radio links to 26 stations, including a few district hospitals and a number of outlying dispensaries, which were equipped with pedal-operated transceivers. The network of dispensaries and hospitals covered a relatively large area, mostly in North-Western State, the distance between the furthest stations being more than 600 kilometres. The dispensaries and hospitals were provided with landing strips for the use of small aircraft.

Two-way radios were used mostly for advising on and supervising the clinical work of the dispensary attendants and for consultation in difficult cases. In the absence of other means of telecommunication, the radios were also used to inform headquarters of shortages of supplies in the dispensaries or possible epidemics in the area. In emergencies an aircraft or other means of transport was requested, to take a doctor to the spot or to move the patient to the hospital.

In the beginning, the project was entirely funded from foreign donations, which also made it possible to purchase two small aircraft for the flying component of the service. This component had to be discontinued later owing to technical and financial difficulties, after which the service functioned only as a two-way radio system. After a few years the scheme was handed over to the Government and was continued through public financing.

During the first years the two-way radio system worked relatively well, but gradually the transceivers aged and became outdated and their maintenance was a great problem. By March 1974 only the base station and a few other transceivers were in working condition, although they were not in operation. Because of the satisfactory performance in the past, the state government is considering the establishment of a radio network with new, modern transceivers in North-Western State.

Results of the scheme

Although the network covered only a small proportion of the dispensaries in the region, including some of the most outlying ones, the two-way radio scheme had the following specific effects, which indicate the potential of such a network in developing countries generally :

1. It provided a means for the further training of the dispensary staff through regular consultations with a doctor. The professional competence, skills, and efficiency of the dispensary staff were thereby increased.

2. It made it possible to supervise the work of the dispensary staff, e.g., by instructing them to devote more of their time to preventive activities, particularly when curative supplies ran short.

3. It enabled the supply of drugs and dressings to be improved and the available supplies to be utilized more efficiently.

4. It enabled many patients, in the dispensaries as well as in the district hospitals, to receive better treatment than they would have had if the system had not existed.

5. It made available better professional advice in emergencies, and often transport to hospital as well.

6. The possibility of direct consultation with a doctor improved the morale of the dispensary staff, who felt less isolated and neglected.

7. Epidemiological surveillance of larger areas was made possible, and in outbreaks of epidemic disease messages reached headquarters rapidly, so that mobile teams could be instructed and dispatched quickly.

Applicability of two-way radios to health services

A two-way radio network is particularly applicable in the following conditions :
— in sparsely populated areas where distances between health posts may be great ;
— in areas where transport conditions are particularly difficult, e.g., through lack of roads or vehicles ;
— in the absence of other adequate telecommunication systems, which may make the use of a radio network feasible even in more densely populated areas with a road network.

Constraints

Experience of the use of two-way radios in Northern Nigeria suggests that certain constraints have to be taken into account in planning and managing a radio network for health services. The most important are as follows :

1. The costs of establishing and maintaining a two-way radio network increase in proportion to the number of radio sets, i.e., in proportion to the number of health institutions to be covered by the radio network. On the other hand, the benefits of the network obviously depend on the coverage provided.

2. As with any technical device, the training of the staff using the radios needs to include an adequate knowledge of the operation and maintenance of the sets.

3. The training of staff needs also to include standard instructions and a terminology to simplify verbal communication by radio.

4. Both the regular servicing and the emergency repair of the radio sets must be well organized.

5. There must be regular supervision of the radio network, with a built-in evaluation scheme.

The cost of establishing a two-way radio network depends mainly on the number of radio sets, i.e., the number of health institutions to be covered by the network. In 1974, a high-frequency radio with a range of 1600 kilometres cost approximately US $1800 with the necessary equipment. The price is somewhat lower for radios with a shorter range. The same type of radio can be used both centrally and peripherally, though a more sophisticated type would be useful at the centre. About US $1000 would cover the basic spare parts for 70 radios, while essential repair tools and other materials to be held at the base would cost approximately US $6000.

The recurrent costs of maintaining a two-way radio network also depend to a large extent on the number of radio sets, although some (e.g., the salary of a radio engineer and assistant) cannot be avoided even with a small number of sets.

It is difficult to measure by cost-benefit analysis the impact of a two-way radio scheme on the health status of a population, though clearly the possibility of consultation can considerably strengthen the services provided by peripheral health units. When a scheme is properly managed and the sets are properly used, recurrent costs may be expected to play a smaller role than capital costs.

III. CONCLUSIONS

In Part I of this report, some aspects of what may be called conventional health services were singled out as factors in the failure of the present systems to meet the basic health needs in developing countries. Part II examines ways of dealing with those factors in the context of some different and apparently successful approaches. From an analysis of the differences brought out by this comparison, a number of conclusions can be drawn.

But first we should ask a preliminary question : have the approaches described been really successful, or are they at least really promising ? In the cases of China and Cuba, a definite positive answer can be given, based largely on statistical and other factual information. In the other cases, as noted in the Introduction, the accounts are based on observational evidence, since health and vital statistics were either unavailable or not significant because of the short lives of the programmes. However, the inevitable subjectivity of the observational method has been balanced as far as possible by field visits, interviews with providers and consumers of health care, discussions with the administrators in charge, and a study of the documents available. All observations were made by panels (whenever possible, multidisciplinary) of experts of varied experience and background, and never by single individuals. In answer to the preliminary question, then, the study may be considered sufficiently accurate and complete to serve as a basis for general conclusions, the most important being that, despite the immense problems and the daunting economic situation, it is possible, using the resources available, to meet certain basic health needs of populations in developing countries, achieve better health care coverage, and improve the levels of health.

The driving force for change

The cases observed belong to two major categories. On the one hand there are programmes adopted nationally, in China, Cuba, Tanzania and, to a certain extent, Venezuela ; on the other, there are schemes covering limited areas, in Bangladesh, India, Niger and Yugoslavia. What characterizes successful national programmes is a strong political will that has transformed a practicable methodology into a national endeavour. In all the countries where this has happened, health has been given a high priority in the government's general development programme. In most cases there has been a fundamental decision to accept substantial changes instead of looking for solutions within the existing system.

Enterprise and leadership are also found in the second group of more limited schemes. Valuable lessons, both technical and operational, can be derived from this type of effort, in spite of its being confined to a limited area. In all cases, the leading role of a dedicated person can be clearly identified. There is also evidence that community leaders and organizations have given considerable support to these projects. External aid has played a part and has apparently been well used. Every effort should be made —although this is one of the most difficult factors for an international body to influence—to pick out the driving forces behind promising programmes and to help harness them to national plans.

Clear national health policies

In most cases changes have led to major shifts of emphasis in the health services—from a curative to a curative-preventive approach, from urban to rural populations, from the privileged to the underprivileged, and from vertical mass campaigns to a system of integrated health services forming a component of overall social and economic development.

Whenever policies to provide health care for the whole population have been put into practice, a standardized and simplified technology has been introduced for primary health care workers to follow as far as possible. Special textbooks for the training of primary health workers and manuals for use in their daily work have proved successful in several countries, for example Cuba, Niger and Venezuela.

In most cases this " deprofessionalization " of technology has been associated with the use of primary health workers with limited, task-oriented training. The front-line health care they provide has been shown to be satisfactory for specified priority health interventions, which are necessarily restricted in range. For this care to continue to be effective and serve its purpose, the health workers need periodic refresher training, supervision and technical advice, and a higher level to which to refer patients. In other words, in order to cover the entire population, the whole health system has to be reoriented to support the primary level.

The health structure has been adjusted in this way as a basic policy, although to different degrees, in all the cases studied. The variations depend on local circumstances or the methods used to carry out the programme. As an example, in Cuba, with its larger numbers of trained personnel, the range of primary care measures is wider than in, say, the Maradi programme in Niger. In both, however, the technology has been modified as much as proved necessary, and both involved changes in other levels of the system to support primary care.

Proper identification of the population's needs and priorities

Although it may seem elementary, the principle of identifying the population's needs and priorities is often neglected in practice., The failure to base action on these needs is often a result of lack of information or sensitivity at the central and local level. In all the cases studied, a conscious effort was made to identify health needs and the underlying causes of poor health, and importance was attached to the needs of the deprived populations (usually in the majority). Particular emphasis was placed on malnutrition and lack of water supply. The systems based on identified needs have a completely different orientation to those copied from developed countries, which often concentrate on privileged minorities. In all the cases in the study, a proper system has been created that enables the people to express their health needs.

Health and development

The health services are only one factor contributing to the health of a population. Economic and social development activities often have a positive influence on a community's health status. Sanitation, housing, nutrition, education and communications are all important factors contributing to good health by improving the quality of life. In their absence, the gains obtainable with the disease-centred machinery of health services cannot go beyond a certain point.

The essence of a successful development programme is that it should be properly balanced. Health services should neither be too sophisticated nor lag behind other sectors in development. Good health must surely be a basic component of economic development; in turn, social and economic development contributes to good health. The relationship is not completely understood, but even partial knowledge can prevent grossly inappropriate sectoral programmes being set up.

In some of the cases studied (e.g., China, Cuba, Tanzania), the health programme has been integrated into a general development programme. In others, it is associated with more limited measures aimed at improving the quality of life.

However, a complete change in the economic and social structure of a country is not the only path to follow. Regional programmes, as in Niger and Venezuela, have shown that less ambitious endeavours can meet basic health needs.

Community involvement

Adequate coverage and use of preventive and curative health services at the village level have been achieved when the population takes major responsibility for primary health care in collaboration with the health services. The principle of local self-reliance implies that local contributions play an important part in providing the necessary manpower and facilities and in bringing the health services into line with needs, wants and priorities of the population they serve. Community involvement also means that the population participates in decision-making about its health services. Participation usually guarantees that community's motivation to accept and use the services, and feeds information on its felt needs and aspirations back to the decision-makers.

Particularly important are the untapped resources within the communities themselves : on the one hand, all the contributions that any community can provide in the shape of facilities, manpower, logistic support, and, possibly, funds ; on the other, the more subtle, but equally important, contribution that people can make by joining in and using the health services. This is particularly true of preventive and protective measures—an essential aspect if the people are to derive the greatest benefit from the limited resources available and if expensive curative care and unnecessary human loss are to be reduced to a minimum.

The need to make use of all the resources available has been recognized in all the cases studied. It is reflected in the common basic policy of involving the community in the responsibility for organizing, orienting, carrying out and in some cases financing primary health care. In China, Tanzania, the Jamkhed area in India, Savar in Bangladesh and Maradi in Niger, local involvement ranges from the selection of primary health workers from among the population to the construction and maintenance of health facilities and help in the financing of the services through population-based payments and other support to the health workers. In many cases, local bodies have been established to help to set priorities and choose between alternative programmes, for example in Jamkhed.

All the approaches employed one or more methods of gaining the understanding, cooperation and support of the population. Political methods relying on party organizations were the most common, but other techniques—for example, the use of development workers or educators—were also shown to be possible. Mass mobilization of the people has proved very effective, especially to achieve readily identifiable goals, such as the campaign against the five pests in China or the mass health education programmes in Tanzania or Ivanjica. In Cuba this method is being used to identify overall health needs and to implement community health programmes.

Reallocation of funds and other resources: a more equitable distribution of funds

In many countries a large proportion of the health resources is expended in a few cities for the benefit of a small proportion of the population. In successful approaches such as China's or Tanzania's, this disproportion is corrected by giving priority in the allocation of funds and personnel to rural areas. In Cuba, with its large urban population, preference is given to clinics serving a large population and to preventive work.

Forms of funding range from almost complete financing by the central government to payment of a considerable share by the community itself. In Venezuela, and in Cuba under a planned economy, the national government has been able to fund primary health care directly. In all other cases, irrespective of the political and economic system, the community has shared this responsibility to a varying degree. The cases show that community sharing of the cost of primary health care or community inputs of other kinds should, together with community participation in the decision-making process, be considered very favourably in designing primary health care systems. Financing and decision-making are complementary functions that reinforce each other ; they place the community in a position of authority as it shoulders responsibility for its own services. In countries where this is the national approach, community leaders are well aware of local health problems. They understand the role, scope and potential of their primary health care service, and they take an active interest in its management. What is more, the health institution at the level nearest to primary care is clearly more alert to the community's needs and wishes.

It was not possible in each case to examine the amount, distribution and utilization of resources within the health structure, but further research on the financing of the delivery of primary health care would obviously be justified.

Manpower development for national health needs

As the shortage of health personnel is one of the main factors preventing the health services from increasing their coverage of the rural areas, the possibility of training health manpower in a different way must be considered seriously. Moreover, if health staff are to be used properly, at the lowest cost, the tasks in the country's various health installations should be defined and the training geared to them. Here the case studies clearly demonstrate certain innovative features.

Primary health workers, locally recruited and supported by their communities, form the front line of the health system and the entry point into it for the population. They are effective, acceptable and inexpensive, and they require only brief initial training. In many of the countries studied, primary health workers are assigned to such priority areas as communicable diseases, maternal and child health (including family planning), nutrition, sanitation, and curative services for minor illness.

Although it is easier to train health workers to perform a specific job rather than multiple tasks, primary health staff of different levels and training were effective in most of the programmes reviewed. Medical assistants, public health nurses and their auxiliaries, barefoot doctors, rural medical aides, family welfare workers and village health workers were found working in rural areas and carrying out diverse functions. At the village level, only some of these health workers were permanently available. In some countries traditional birth attendants were taught elementary skills and given enough basic knowledge to become part of the government health system.

The experience of China has shown that indigenous healers can be trained and integrated in the general health system. Indigenous systems of health care function among large populations in the developing world, and in some countries, such as India, the system is well established although unrecognized. Further integration of these indigenous practitioners—professionals, nonprofessionals, faith healers, magic healers—into the state system calls for more research and information.

100

Dr. Sanka thea
Sri Lanka

- Trust only curative work
- In prophylatric Rx, they do a good job
- Confidence of the people

Botswana Survey —

If the approach to health is multisectoral, workers from other sectors, for example community development workers or teachers, can be associated with a health programme, as in Tanzania and Jamkhed.

Supervision and in-service training are the responsibility of staff at the intermediate level, who need special understanding, knowledge and skills in order to work with and train primary health workers and indigenous practitioners. In China, in order to see local conditions and problems at first hand, the supervisory staff work in rural areas at regular intervals. Systems for the continuous training of primary health workers have been set up in China, Cuba, Venezuela and the Jamkhed project in India.

Decentralization of planning and administration

A central authority that merely hands decisions down to lower levels does not stimulate sufficient local participation. The planning process is inevitably changed when the local population is involved in making the decisions.

Of the countless ways of reorganizing the planning and administrative machinery, several examples are provided by the case studies. All the national alternatives exhibit the general characteristic of a national body that sets policy and decides on requests, coupled with a means of channelling information on needs and wants to it from the periphery.

The development of a decentralized system is undoubtedly one of the most difficult undertakings facing a country trying to improve its people's health. It can be reasonably argued that the result is not worth the effort and that a completely centralized system is more efficient. The best answer to the argument, though a limited one, is to be found in the case studies, which show that the most impressive gains have been made in countries where a strong central policy has been implemented by a decentralized executive organization. The degree of decentralization differs from one case to another, varying from complete managerial devolution to the community (China) to a redistribution of responsibilities within the health system accompanied by consultation with communities (Venezuela).

Examples of community participation are found in different political settings. Participation makes communities more readily mobilized, increases their health awareness, and provides health authorities with the information they need for a better and more sensitive administration.

Integration and coordination

Two kinds of integration are evident in the case studies. The first is the integration of the various aspects of health policy into economic and social development. Joint action is pursued with such sectors as education, agriculture, public works, housing and communications, particularly at the local level and with the participation of the community. Examples are Ivanjica, Jamkhed and the Jurain applied nutrition project in Bangladesh. Tanzania, as part of its rural development policy, is consolidating the rural population into larger settlements, which makes it easier to provide primary health and other services and minimizes one of the worst problems for rural health services in many developing countries, that of distance.

The second kind of integration is the welding of the different parts of the health services into a national whole (maternal and child care, family planning, prevention of communicable diseases, nutrition, health education, etc.). This has been done, for example, in Bangladesh. The main practical feature of this type of integration is the retraining of field workers from mass campaigns for more general health purposes.

Health and nutrition education

In all the approaches studied, without exception, health education is one of the main activities of primary health care. This understanding of the importance of health education has been responsible for a large share of the success achieved by China and promises success in other programmes. Since health education has been a deplorable failure in conventional health services, the strategy followed in these successful instances merits careful consideration.

In Savar and Jurain, Bangladesh, health education is pursued on a vast scale and also forms part of training activities in agriculture and other sectors apart from health. Associated with community participation, it has already produced a distinct change in the people's attitude to health and the health services. Family planning has also made substantial gains. In Jurain, most of the improvements in nutrition practices can be related in one way or another to the major educational drive launched there.

Success in spreading health education seems to rest on several factors. The association of development programmes with mobilization and participation of the people is in itself a most important means of stimulating health awareness in a community. Participation by the community in decision-making, if assisted by trained personnel aware of the actual and felt needs of the people, can also be a powerful force in education. In the most successful cases, the educational message was carried by workers who belonged to the community and hence enjoyed its confidence and shared the same views, aspirations and " language ". The message they transmitted was generally simple and dealt with the most important problems.

Sanitation

All the programmes studied emphasized the importance of providing basic sanitation for rural areas, and particularly a supply of safe water. In Tanzania both the Government and the local authorities have given high priority to a rural water supply system, while the Jamkhed project stresses a scheme for the drilling of irrigation wells.

Ministries of health have limited scope for action in the field of sanitation, which is usually the domain of other government agencies. Many of the projects undertaken by water resource, housing and town planning agencies and ministries of agriculture and education have considerable potential for improving health that can often be realized at little additional cost if the health component is integrated into the project at the planning stage.

Major water, sewage and other sanitary engineering schemes are clearly a government responsibility, but many rural projects can be tackled by local authorities and planned and carried out by local community organizations, as has been done in China, Cuba, Tanzania, Ivanjica, and Jamkhed.

Communication and transport

Serious thought should be given to ways of delivering health services with less dependence on mechanical transport (powered by petrol or diesel fuel) than at present. Motor vehicles reserved for the exclusive use of health services are expensive to run and maintain. Public transport is often available to satisfy part of the need. In the face of constantly rising operating costs, greater use could be made of bicycles, small motorcycles and other more economical traditional forms of transport. Sharing rides will make better use of existing transport and reduce the need for extra vehicles. However, in the supervision of primary health services quick and reliable transport is necessary to provide effective guidance and technical advice.

Modern technology offers many possibilities of improving communications. Although there have been some experiments in the application of new means of communication to rural health services, the techniques have not been fully explored. There has been a tendency to focus on some of the more expensive types of transport while other means of communication have been relatively neglected.

For example, two-way radios, forming communication links between primary health workers in remote areas and consultants and supervisors in medical centres, appear to have promise, but their use may be limited by the initial investment required, the operating cost, and the lack of maintenance and repair facilities. Factors like these need to be taken into account when new schemes are considered.

It may be possible to make greater use for health purposes of communication and transport schemes developed for the police, national broadcasting or other government activities.

Summary of the conclusions

A firm national policy of providing health care for the underprivileged will involve a virtual revolution in most health service systems. It will bring about changes in the distribution of power, in the pattern of political decision-making, in the attitude and commitment of the health professionals and administrators in ministries of health and universities, and in people's awareness of what they are entitled to. To achieve such far-reaching changes, political leaders will have to shoulder the responsibility of overcoming the inertia or opposition of the health professions and other well-entrenched vested interests.

Fundamental changes in health care of this kind in the developing countries will require correspondingly far-reaching changes in the organizational structure and management practices of the health services. For illustrative purposes three different types of health delivery systems, appropriate to the differing stages of a country's development and relying heavily on primary health workers, are outlined in Annex 2. Although many variations of these three types are possible, such services need to be manned by a new brand of health professional with a wider social outlook, trained to respond to the actual requirements of the population. The basis and the strength of such services lie in a cadre of suitably trained primary health workers chosen by the people from among themselves and controlled by them, rather than in a reluctant, alienated, frustrated group of bureaucrats " parachuted " into the community. The entire health service system will need to be mobilized to strengthen and support these primary health workers by providing them with training, supervision, referral facilities and logistic support, including a simplified national health technology appropriate to their needs. Primary health services of this kind will also function in close coordination with other segments of the health services and with other services that have a bearing on the health status of the masses, such as education, agriculture, public works and social welfare.

The innovations and successes described in this study are sufficiently promising to warrant a major change in policy and direction enabling such programmes to be fostered, extended, adapted and used as examples for a large-scale global programme.

IV. RECOMMENDATIONS TO WHO AND UNICEF

The health care delivery systems that were taken as examples for this study show characteristics that appear to have been instrumental in leading to wider and more evenly distributed primary health care, greater satisfaction for the consumers, and more effective and more economical delivery of services. Properly adapted, these systems appear to be applicable in many political, social, economic and environmental situations.

The following recommendations [a] are accordingly made to the governing bodies of WHO and UNICEF, although by the nature of the subject some of the recommendations may be considered as addressed also to governments.

(1) WHO and UNICEF should adopt an action programme aimed at extending primary health care to populations in developing countries, particularly to those which are now inadequately provided with such care, such as rural and remote populations, slum dwellers and nomads. Since the development of primary health care services is a national undertaking that requires action at all levels, and since it is hardly feasible for all countries to introduce radical reforms, the proposed action programme should initially be selective. The criteria for selection should include one or more of the following : (i) the existence of a national decision to proceed along this path ; (ii) a potential for change ; or (iii) local health endeavours which could lead at a later step to national change.

(2) The following principles in the reorientation and development of health services to achieve extensive primary care should be adopted subject to local conditions :

(a) primary health care services should be recognized as forming part of overall development (of urban, rural and other underserved groups), taking into account the interaction between development and health programmes ;

(b) firm policies, priorities and plans should be established for the proposed primary health services ;

(c) all other levels of the health system should be reoriented to provide support (referral, training, advisory, supervisory and logistic) to the primary health care level. Such an orientation of the health system would require active participation and training in the basic principles for all members of the health services ;

(d) communities should be involved in the designing, staffing and functioning of their local primary health care centres, and in other forms of support ;

(e) primary health care workers who have undergone simple training should be utilized ;

(f) the primary health care workers should be selected, when possible, by the community itself, or at least in consultation with the community— acceptability of such workers is in fact a crucial factor of success ;

(g) there should be special emphasis on (i) preventive measures ; (ii) health and nutrition education ; (iii) health care needs of mothers

---

[a] As approved by the UNICEF/WHO Joint Committee on Health Policy in February 1975 and included in the report on its twentieth session (WHO Official Records, No. 228, 1975, Annex 2).

and children ; (iv) utilization of simplified forms of medical and health technology ; (v) association with some traditional forms of health care and use of traditional practitioners ; and (vi) respect for the cultural patterns and felt needs in health and community development of the consumers.

(3) A programme proposal such as that recommended requires a detailed awareness and understanding by all members of WHO and UNICEF staff and an organizational adaptation to respond to the new challenges. Therefore it is recommended that positive planned steps should be taken by WHO and UNICEF to inform, educate, and orient their staffs to these policies.

(4) WHO and UNICEF should study in detail not only the innovations described in this study but also those that are occurring continuously in different parts of the world under different sponsorship ; they should record and monitor them ; learn from them ; evaluate them ; make their results widely available ; assist them when necessary ; adapt them ; build upon them ; and encourage similar endeavours, even though some may present some risk in the sense that their favourable outcome is not clearly predictable. Some of these risks can be minimized by adequate preparation and the building of a meaningful partnership with government.

(5) WHO and UNICEF should pursue research on the effects of rural and community development of the health of people and on the role that other sectors can play in the delivery of primary health care, develop methodology for application of the findings, and assist in its implementation.

(6) WHO and UNICEF should encourage and support :

(a) the adaptation of manpower planning and educational methods and techniques to situations in developing countries ;

(b) the introduction of changes in the curricula and training of doctors, nurses and midwives to enable them to discharge their duties as envisaged in a health service system oriented towards primary health care ;

(c) the introduction of changes in the training programmes of other health personnel to provide community orientation and inculcate the health team concept, so that such personnel become integral members of the community capable of putting the local resources available to the best use.

(7) Within the context of national resources and plans, WHO and UNICEF should seek the definition and adaptation of medical and health technology so that primary health workers can use as much of it as possible.

(8) WHO and UNICEF should study promising existing or potential approaches in health education with a view to disseminating knowledge

about them and sponsoring their application, so as to create health awareness in people and encourage them to become partners in the delivery of primary health care.

(9) WHO and UNICEF should study possible solutions to transport and communications difficulties in the delivery of primary health services and should encourage the implementation of promising solutions, particularly in rural areas.

(10) The comments of national health administrations should be solicited, for use in the development of plans of operations.

(11) The report on the joint study should be widely circulated among international organizations and in developing countries, particularly among those responsible for the formulation of national policies, plans and programmes affecting the health of populations in rural and other under-privileged areas. An edited version might subsequently be published.

ACKNOWLEDGEMENTS

The contributions of the following persons to this study are greatly appreciated: the representatives of the governments of the countries visited; the more than 80 experts throughout the world who contributed through their papers; Dr K. Newell, Dr P. Fazzi, and Dr R. H. O. Bannerman (WHO); Dr C. Egger, Mr N. Bowles, and Dr G. Sicault (UNICEF); Professor E. Brown, Professor R. Giglio, and Professor M. Roemer; members of the consultation held in the summer of 1974—Dr A. Adeniyi-Jones, Dr D. Banerji, Dr E. K. Chagula, Dr G. J. Ebrahim, Dr N. R. E. Fendall, Dr D. Ferguson, Dr C. L. Gonzalez, Dr S. Haraldson, and Dr V. W. Sidel; members of the steering committee drawn from the staff of UNICEF and WHO; and staff of Headquarters and Regional Offices, the field staff, and the country representatives of the two Organizations who assisted in the study.

Annex 1

WHO AND UNICEF POLICIES

WHO's policy on basic health services

As early as 1951, at a time when many developing countries were concentrating their efforts on specialized mass campaigns for the eradication of diseases, the Director-General of WHO stated in his annual report [a] that these efforts would have only temporary results if they were not followed by the establishment of permanent health services in rural areas to deal with the day-to-day work in the control and prevention of disease and the promotion of health.

In 1953 the WHO Executive Board, in a resolution later endorsed by the Sixth World Health Assembly, stated that " assistance in the health field [financed by the United Nations Expanded Programme of Technical Assistance] should be designed primarily to strengthen the basic health service of the country and to meet the most urgent problems affecting large sections of the population, with due regard to the stage of social or economic development of the country concerned ".[b]

While providing support for the malaria and smallpox eradication programmes as well as campaigns to control various communicable diseases, the Executive Board and the Health Assembly have since repeatedly re-affirmed the importance of improving and extending basic health services. A number of expert committees, particularly those on public health administration, made statements to the same effect between 1952 and 1960.[c] Nevertheless, achievements have remained modest, falling far short of needs.

During the 1960s the policy of promoting basic health services, by then more clearly defined, began to influence some developing countries. In 1962, the Fifteenth World Health Assembly recognized that " while it is normally necessary for a malaria eradication programme to be implemented by a specialized service, the active participation of the health service assumes considerable importance as the programme progresses towards its goal, becoming fundamental in the maintenance phase when vigilance against the re-establishment of the infection becomes the responsibility of health services ".[d]

---

[a] WHO Official Records, No. 38, 1952, p. 2.

[b] *Handbook of Resolutions and Decisions*, Vol. I, 1948–1972, pp. 245–246, resolutions EB11.R57.6 and WHA6.27.

[c] WHO Technical Report Series, No. 428, 1969 (*The organization and administration of maternal and child health services*: fifth report of the WHO Expert Committee on Maternal and Child Health).

[d] *Handbook of Resolutions and Decisions*, Vol. I, 1948–1972, p. 75, resolution WHA15.19.

108

The next few years saw increasing recognition of the desirability of integrating special programmes with basic health services. The UNICEF/ WHO Joint Committee on Health Policy confirmed this approach at its session in 1965.

This trend in the Organization's policy has grown stronger in the successive general programmes of work covering a specific period. In the first programme of work (1952–1955),[a] it was stated that projects in specialized fields should be a stage towards the ultimate goal of a balanced and integrated health programme. In the second (1957–1960),[b] the concept of the importance of developing the rural health services appeared. This concept was clarified and developed in the third general programme (1962–1965),[c] adopted in 1960 : " WHO has sponsored campaigns against specific diseases and has promoted specialized services. It is probable that within the next five years governments will seek the assistance of WHO in converting these campaigns and services into more integrated programmes and the Organization should be ready to provide this assistance ". The fourth programme (1967–1971) [d] went further, stating that " experience has shown that for the success of mass campaigns it has been frequently necessary to assimilate their machinery, with the limited objectives, into the more comprehensive general health service, which at times had to be developed for the purpose. This integration of the mass campaign organization within the general health services facilitates the extension of those services to the peripheral areas of a country, and avoids the centralization which tends to prevent progress in territories with rural characteristics and a scattered distribution of population ". In the fifth general programme of work (1973–1977),[e] adopted in 1971, it was stated that the concepts of integration and development of basic health services should pervade the entire programme. Over the years the basic health services have come to be accorded considerable importance and to be assigned priority in country health programmes. Principles for the establishment and development of national health systems were set out by the Twenty-third World Health Assembly in 1970.[f]

In 1971, the Twenty-fourth Health Assembly asked the Executive Board to carry out an organizational study on " Methods of promoting the development of basic health services ".[g] Two years later, on the basis of

---

a WHO Official Records, No. 32, 1951, Annex 10.
b WHO Official Records, No. 63, 1955, Annex 4.
c WHO Official Records, No. 102, 1960, Annex 2.
d WHO Official Records, No. 143, 1965, Annex 3.
e WHO Official Records, No. 193, 1971, Annex 11.
f Handbook of Resolutions and Decisions, Vol. I, 1948–1972, pp. 29–30, resolution WHA23.61.
g Ibid., p. 483, resolution WHA24.38.

this study, the Health Assembly reiterated its " strong conviction that each Member State should develop a health service that is both accessible and acceptable to the total population, suited to its needs and to the socio-economic conditions of the country, and at the level of health technology considered necessary to meet the problems of that country at a given time ".[a]

In line with these policies, the number of WHO projects in all regions directly related to basic health services increased from 85 in 1965 to 156 in 1971. During the same period, over and above the projects, a considerable number of courses, seminars, symposia and technical discussions related to the development of basic health services were held in all continents, while research was carried out on the organization of community health services.

Despite these statements of policy and modifications of the Organization's programme the 20 years between 1951 and 1971 did not show convincingly that the present course of action by WHO or by most countries will bring a solution to the problems within a reasonable period. In its organizational study on the development of basic health services, the Executive Board concluded that the present position is unsatisfactory. The joint WHO/UNICEF study provides a further opportunity to take stock and to propose amended approaches, policies and action.

UNICEF's assistance policy

For nearly 25 years a major part of UNICEF's resources has been channelled through the organized health services in developing countries. From 1970 to 1974, assistance to child health represented 51% of all UNICEF programme aid. At present, UNICEF is assisting health services for children in 99 countries. It was realized from the beginning that neither the countries nor UNICEF had the means to provide medical care and treatment for every child in these countries ; thus, while its aid focused on support for national maternal and child health services, UNICEF also gave considerable attention to indirect or protective measures. In all these activities, UNICEF has worked in close partnership with WHO.

Through maternal and child health services, concern was first centred on prenatal, obstetrical and postnatal care. More recently—in the past 10 years or so—UNICEF has become increasingly concerned with the young child after weaning up to the age of five years and has sought to reinforce services to this age group through maternal and child health centres. Since 1967, it has also assisted family planning.

Since its inception, UNICEF has thrown its weight behind mass campaigns designed to control diseases seriously affecting children, including tuberculosis, leprosy, yaws and malaria. It has provided sub-stantial aid for the production of vaccines and sera in many countries, and

---

[a] WHO Official Records, No. 209, 1973, p. 18, resolution WHA26.35.

has assisted environmental sanitation programmes emphasizing water supply on a pilot or demonstration scale in rural areas.

In all these activities, UNICEF has given high priority to assisting the training of local personnel in their own countries. It devotes about one-third of its aid to helping to establish and strengthen training institutions and schemes at all levels—planning, directing, teaching, supervisory, auxiliary and volunteer. Major emphasis is placed on the training of middle-level and primary health personnel. UNICEF believes that, in training, more attention needs to be given to local conditions, to the preparation of trainers, to supervision and to the local production of suitable teaching aids.

From the first, although urban maternal and child health services were not excluded, UNICEF directed most of the assistance to rural areas.

In the course of time, it was realized that maternal and child health services could function best in the context of and with the support of broad national health services, and UNICEF assistance was extended to those elements of the broad services that support and supplement services for the mother and child. It was recognized that child health must be seen as part of the health of the community as a whole.

At the same time, as mass campaigns progressed towards their goal of bringing specific diseases under control, it became evident that some sort of permanent establishment was necessary to maintain the benefits gained. Vertical mass campaigns should clearly not be continued indefinitely but should be integrated into the regular health services. Although UNICEF has supported the integration of mass campaigns into basic health services and substantial progress has been made, the limited coverage of health networks has posed a serious problem.

UNICEF aid for child nutrition, which first took the form of supplementary child feeding and aid to local dairies, began to expand in range in the mid-1950s with the development of low-cost protein-rich food mixtures. UNICEF also began aiding " applied nutrition " programmes through such channels as community development, agricultural extension, schools and health services so as to stimulate and help the rural population to grow and eat the foods it required for better child nutrition. More recently, FAO, UNICEF and WHO have been encouraging the development of national food and nutrition policies that make provision for child nutrition.

After the mid-1950s, programmes in primary education, social welfare and applied nutrition in which UNICEF took part showed that the activities of health services should be combined with activities in other fields such as education, social welfare and agricultural extension.

This led to a major change in UNICEF's basic policy, which was confirmed by its Executive Board in 1964. At that time, UNICEF recognized that a sectoral approach to the needs of and services for children was not satisfactory. Two main recommendations were made, in which governments were invited to undertake national interdisciplinary surveys in order to :

(1) identify the basic needs of children ; and (2) elaborate national policies for children and youth so as to harmonize and coordinate all sectoral activities for the young. It was emphasized that child health should not be seen in isolation from the total needs of children ; rather, their needs and development must be seen as a whole and as a continuing process. Because children are not simply the recipients of services, but valuable assets in national growth and development, policies and programmes for them should be worked out in the context of national development plans, maternal and child health services finding their place in the broad national perspective.

Within this multisectoral approach, UNICEF has reemphasized the role of basic health services, together with improvement in water supplies, alleviation of the work of women, and special attention to the young child and deprived population groups.

DIFFERENT TYPES OF HEALTH SERVICES ADAPTED
TO DIFFERENT DEGREES OF DEVELOPMENT

The different types of health delivery systems outlined below are intended to be illustrative only and should not be considered as patterns of health services recommended by WHO and UNICEF. Obviously, many variations of these three levels of health services are possible.

1. *The simplest type—at the peripheral level*

Village health posts

(a) *Selected tasks*

Elementary services for mother and children—deliveries by traditional birth attendants ; promotional measures in relation to nutrition and immunization ;
Elementary sanitation—such as protection of wells, waste disposal, food protection, vector control ;
Simple health education ;
Rule-of-thumb procedures for managing easily recognizable diseases and symptom complexes ; about 10–15 drugs ;
Participation in immunization programmes ;
Simplest family planning and health education.

(b) *Manpower*

Local persons selected by the villagers, with primary education wherever possible and trained as far as possible in an in-service situation ;
Traditional birth attendants given a short basic training and refresher instruction at twice-yearly seminars.

(c) *Community participation*

Provision of a room or small health post ;
Maintenance of the room or building ;
Payment of part of the salary of the health worker ;
Transport of patients referred elsewhere ;
Simple sanitation such as protection of wells, waste disposal, food protection and vector/vermin control, if possible working with the teacher or extension worker for sanitation, health education or food production, and the community development organizer ;

Food storage and protection from vermin, fungi, damp or other spoilage.

(d) *Supervision (educative role)*

One primary health worker with one-year training, or less if compensated by at least two years' experience.

(e) *Transport*

None ; or ox-cart, simple bicycle, or public transport.

(f) *Equipment*

Very simple : table, chairs, 10–15 selected drugs ;
UNICEF midwife kits (with contents periodically reviewed) ;
Labour-saving devices (pumps, wheelbarrows, bicycle, trailers, grain mills, simple tools).

(g) *Referral centres*

Simple—staffed by primary health workers or medical assistants.

(h) *Particular cases*

For scattered populations, ambulatory services with one auxiliary or one medical assistant coming once a week to the local village centres.
Nomadic populations—one member of the tribe trained (who could be provided with an identification card to be accepted by the health services).

2. *Intermediate type*

(a) *Selected tasks*

Same as in section 1 (a), plus :
Family planning ;
Nutritional education (including distribution of vitamins, protective foods and weaning foods) ; special attention should be paid to local sources of vitamins ;
Immunizations ;
Detection of cases (surveillance activities following mass eradication campaigns) ;
Food production, conservation and storage ;
Cooperation with other sectors (agriculture, education, general development).

(b) *Manpower*

One primary health worker with primary school background, plus :
Local recruitment of volunteers ;
Traditional practitioners (including traditional birth attendants).

(c) *Participation of the community*

Same as in section 1 (c), plus :
Community involvement through cooperation of the village community and local government services, namely

— local chiefs,

— teachers and agricultural extension workers,

— promoters (if any),

— social leaders, such as heads of youth or women's associations or local organizations.

(d) *Supervision*

One medical assistant or an experienced primary health worker—if possible a team.

(e) *Communications/transport*

Transport to the referral centre for emergency cases ; for supervision, the cheapest effective use of telephone or two-way radio, if possible.

(f) *Equipment*

A little more elaborate than shown in section 1 (f).

(g) *Referral centre*

Health centre with four beds and transport, staffed by a medical assistant ; oriented towards public health.

3. *More advanced type*

(a) *Selected tasks*

Same as in section 1 (a), plus :
Family planning with auxiliary medical supervision ;
Curative work plus ambulatory treatment of tuberculosis ;
Rehydration for young children ;
Nutritional supplementation : locally produced food, processed food, or mixture ;

Rehabilitation nutrition centres ;
Sanitation, including water, wastes disposal, home improvement ;
School health, etc. ;
Health education ;
Consumer education ;
Insurance schemes.

(b) *Manpower*

A team with :
One medical assistant or traditional doctor and/or primary health
worker ;
One or two locally recruited staff, including an auxiliary midwife
with a minimum of 6–12 months' training.

(c) *Participation of the community*

Same as in section 2 (c), plus :
Cooperative for purchasing and distributing fertilizers ;
Cooperatives for purchasing and distributing selected grains.

(d) *Supervision*

Teams, including public health doctor or medical assistant,
experienced midwife and sanitarian.

(e) *Communications/transport*

Telephone or radio ;
Transport to the referral centre (car or ambulance).

(f) *Equipment*

More elaborate—for diagnosis and treatment, drugs, etc.

(g) *Referral centres*

Rural hospital with certain specialties, including surgery ;
Reference health centres with technicians (laboratory).

In the case of type 3, decentralized planning at the regional, district or
subdistrict level will make it possible to carry out surveys and research,
particularly nutritional surveys.

———